Robert Kowalski is an internationally-acclaimed medical journalist. At the age of 35, Robert had already had a heart attack and bypass surgery and then had further bypass surgery six years later. Because of this he decided to find out everything he could about heart disease. The diet and some of the natural remedies he found out about led him to write his bestselling book *The 8-Week Cholesterol Cure* in 1987. He lives in California.

D0513155

My father passed away on 5 December 1969 from a massive heart attack. Hypertension was one of the major factors contributing to the disease that claimed his life and took him away from us for ever. Oh, how I wish I could have had more time with him. How I wish he could have met my wife and my children, his grandchildren.

I love him. I miss him. And I hope this book that I dedicate to his memory will help others live and beat cardiovascular disease, so they can enjoy the years that were taken away from him by a disease we're learning more and more about every day.

Isobel

8 Weeks
to Lower Blood
Pressure

Take the pressure off your heart without the
use of prescription drugs

Robert E Kowalski

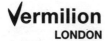

Vermilion
LONDON

1 3 5 7 9 10 8 6 4 2

First published as *Take the Pressure off Your Heart* in Australia by
New Holland Publishers in 2006

Published in 2007 by Vermilion, an imprint of Ebury Publishing
A Random House Group company

Copyright © Robert E Kowalski

Robert E Kowalski has asserted his right to be identified as the author of
this Work in accordance with the Copyright, Designs and Patents
Act 1988

All rights reserved. No part of this publication may be reproduced,
stored in a retrieval system, or transmitted in any form or by any means,
electronic, mechanical, photocopying, recording or otherwise, without
the prior permission of the copyright owner

The Random House Group Limited Reg. No. 954009

Addresses for companies within the Random House Group can be found at
www.randomhouse.co.uk

A CIP catalogue record for this book is available from the British Library

The Random House Group Limited makes every effort to ensure that the
papers used in our books are made from trees that have been legally
sourced from well-managed and credibly certified forests. Our paper
procurement policy can be found on www.randomhouse.co.uk

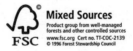

Mixed Sources
Product group from well-managed
forests and other controlled sources
www.fsc.org Cert no. TT-COC-2139
© 1996 Forest Stewardship Council
FSC

Printed and bound in Great Britain by
Mackays of Chatham plc, Chatham, Kent

ISBN 9780091917302

Copies are available at special rates for bulk orders.
Contact the sales development team on 020 7840 8487 or visit
www.booksforpromotions.co.uk for more information.

To buy books by your favourite authors and register for offers, visit
www.rbooks.co.uk

Contents

Acknowledgements

It would be impossible to list every person who helped me write this book and bring it to publication. So I would like to take this opportunity to thank those who assisted with the research process, finding obscure little facts and details, those who reviewed chapters to make sure I was on target scientifically and medically, and those who inspired me to write the book in the first place.

I have deep gratitude to those hundreds and thousands of medical researchers all over the world who continue to add pieces to the jigsaw puzzle of cardiovascular disease. In the months that it took to write and edit this book, there was not a single week that went by that didn't provide an additional insight through a report of a conference I read on the internet or an article or editorial in one of the many journals I read regularly. Most of those men and women don't know me and probably have never heard of me or my books or my personal fight against heart disease. But each has touched me very personally and helped me to share their information with my readers.

My thanks go specifically to those who took their valuable time to review chapters including Steven Burstein, MD, who graciously wrote the foreword to the book and Joseph Keenan, MD, of the University of Minnesota, who has also worked with me in a number of my previous efforts. Thanks also to Douglas Walsh, DO, and his son Douglas Walsh, Jr, DO, a family doctor and internist, respectively, in Florida, who spent their time sharing with me their insights in treating men and women with high blood pressure in the real world outside of university medical centres.

Special thanks to my agent, my publicist and, most importantly, my very good friend, Margaret Gee, for her unflagging support and confidence in my work. I would send her chapters as I completed them, and she quickly responded with her kind words of encouragement.

And, last but far from least, my deep appreciation to Julia Kellaway at Vermilion for bringing this important, potentially life-saving information to the men and women of the United Kingdom.

Foreword

I had the pleasure of meeting Bob Kowalski in 2004 at the recommendation of Dr Jack Sternlieb, a mutual friend and esteemed cardiac surgeon as well as founder of the Heart Institute of the Desert, in Rancho Mirage, California. Bob's medical history had been well characterised. He suffered myocardial infarction (heart attack) at the age of 35, in 1978, had three-vessel bypass surgery later that same year, then required four-vessel bypass surgery in 1984. Despite this overwhelming burden and genetic predisposition, Bob has done exceptionally well over the last 22 years. With great determination and unending intellectual curiosity, Bob has developed a programme applicable for all who wish to prevent, and treat patients at risk of, cardiovascular disease.

Bob Kowalski, an internationally acclaimed medical journalist of more than 28 years, published *The 8-Week Cholesterol Cure*, in April 1987, and a complete revision, *The New 8-Week Cholesterol Cure*, in 2002. He was kind enough to provide me with a copy during one of our initial encounters and I was immediately captivated by his easily understood but comprehensive writing style, which appeals to both the lay and medically educated reader alike. Bob's perspective is interesting in that he not only writes as an authority in his field but also one who continues to battle cardiovascular disease himself on a daily basis. A testament to his approach is the fact that he has defied statistics. One would have quoted him a ten-year survival at the age of 35, having undergone three-vessel heart bypass surgery in 1978. We are thankful that Bob continues to beat the odds as he relentlessly questions medical dogma, educates and pioneers new approaches to disease management.

Bob Kowalski encourages medically trained professionals to think 'outside the box'. We tend to be poorly educated in the non-pharmacologic management of disease. As a group, we are often arrogant, dispelling theories and approaches that we are not comfortable with and criticising them in the name of good medical science. In the UK a huge sum is spent each year on herbal medicines and other alternative treatments. Additionally, this market continues to grow as it is tremendously appealing to patients who are able to manage diseases naturally without hard-core pharmaceuticals. It is therefore our duty as healthcare professionals to be educated in non-traditional 'neutraceuticals' (nutritional supplements with pharmaceutical properties) so that we may both understand and better treat our patients. Bob encourages us to do this by presenting clear and concise data.

As a patient, one can only follow Mr Kowalski's example. He always encourages one to obtain information, educate oneself, fully understand doctors' recommendations and, most importantly, work hand in hand and honestly with your medical professional.

If one were to design an ideal patient, that would be Bob Kowalski. Bob strides through life, savouring the moments, always considering his glass half full. His enthusiasm is infectious and he is a true delight to interact with. A very compliant patient, as long as the recommendations make sense. Always questioning, always seeking out a better alter-native, if possible. With the same gusto and verve, Bob has undertaken another enormous project, that being the comprehensive management of high blood pressure or hyper-tension. This educational tour will take the readers through the history of hypertension, its diagnosis, recommendations for management and contemporary therapies. But more, Bob will present the holistic approach to hypertension and have both patients and doctors understand novel, natural and alternative supplements that can, in many instances, negate the necessity for traditional or hard-core pharmaceuticals. Anecdotally, many doctors have seen patients who have responded exceptionally well to lifestyle modification, exercise, weight loss and moderation in alcohol intake. Supplements such as arginine and grape seed extract have been noted to cure hypertension in my practice. These patients are very proud that they have not had to rely on traditional medications to cure their problem. An advocate and a participant in wonderful doctor-patient relationships, Bob will be able to guide you, the reader, to a healthier and happier life.

Listen and learn from a man with considerable personal experience who speaks not from anecdote but from personal triumph. Bob's advice is succinct and logical, and his recommendations are very doable. This book will educate and motivate, as it has done for me. And let's all remember Bob's quote, 'You can fight heart disease and win.'

Steven Burstein, MD
Associate Director
Cardiac Catheterization Laboratories
Good Samaritan Hospital
Associate Professor of Medicine
UCLA Medical School
Los Angeles, California

Introduction

Suppose you had a crystal ball to see into the future of your health. Let's say that your crystal ball foretold not only the likelihood of major, possibly fatal illnesses but also ways to prevent those problems. Would you take a look? Would you take the steps – especially if they were pretty simple – to avoid those health problems? Most people would. After all, we want the best possible health and the longest, healthiest lives.

I'm one of the very lucky ones. I survived a heart attack and bypass surgery in 1978 at the age of 35 and a second bypass in 1984 at the age of 41. In a very real way, I did have that crystal ball, but I just didn't know how to use it back then. My major risk factor was a high cholesterol level. I'd known that for years before the heart attack, but in those days the issue of cholesterol and heart disease was controversial. Moreover, there weren't effective ways to get cholesterol down to healthy levels.

Interestingly, as the years have gone by, we've learned that the lower we can get our cholesterol counts, the more we slash the risk of developing heart disease. American medical students in the 1950s learned that 'normal' cholesterol levels were a person's age plus 200mg/dL (UK equivalent 5.2mmol/l). It wasn't until the late 1980s that doctors were advising patients to get those levels down to below 200. And today we know that, when it comes to cholesterol, the lower the better.

But this isn't a book about cholesterol, although I'll discuss that issue in one of the chapters. This book deals with another one of the 'Big Three' risk factors for heart attack and stroke

– blood pressure. The third one, by the way, is cigarette smoking. Those three are responsible for the vast majority of heart attacks and strokes, although other factors, especially diabetes, come into play as well.

Ironically, the medical community formally recognised the importance of blood pressure, in 1972, long before that of cholesterol, in 1987. But, as with cholesterol, medical researchers have found, only rather recently, that, for the most part, the lower the better. You can expect that blood pressure control, and prevention of high blood pressure, medically termed 'hypertension', will get increasing attention in the coming years.

The statistics are staggering. Hypertension is the commonest disease treated in general practice in Britain. The 1998 Health Survey for England found that 37 per cent of adults over 16 years of age had blood pressure levels greater than 140/90 mmHG, placing them at increased risk of heart attack and stroke. Cardiovascular disease accounts for about a third of all deaths in the United Kingdom. And both individual doctors and health organisations have put increased emphasis on controlling raised levels of blood pressure (hypertension).

One-third – 65 million – of Americans over the age of 18 have at least mild hypertension. For African-American women, it's half the population and for black men it's a major problem as well. At least one-third of those with high blood pressure are not being treated. That means millions and millions of men and women are at risk. Numbers previously considered normal in the US are now given the new designation 'pre-hypertension'. Since 2003, doctors there have used that term to denote patients whose seemingly okay blood pressure levels predict problems at a later date. There's our crystal ball again. We can predict confidently those who will develop full-blown hypertension in the years to come. Similarly, new joint guidelines published in 2005 by six UK professional societies expanded the criteria for prevention of cardiovascular disease and stroke in primary care.

Researchers at Boston University reported on participants in a study of people under 65 years of age with optimum, normal and high-normal blood pressure, over a four-year period. Of these, 5.3 per cent, 17.6 per cent and 37.3 per cent respectively developed hypertension. For those over 65, the likelihood was 16 per cent, 25.5 per cent and 49.5 per cent respectively. And a mere 5 per cent weight gain jacked up the risk of developing hypertension by an additional 20 to 30 per cent.

The higher one's blood pressure (BP), the greater the risk of heart attack and stroke. That risk is multiplied by additional factors including family history, raised cholesterol levels, diabetes, cigarette smoking, sedentary behaviour, overweight and obesity, diabetes and other considerations. To make matters worse, high BP appears to increase the risk of developing Alzheimer's disease in later life.

I'm no doubt more aware than most people of cardio-vascular disease, a term that lumps together all diseases of the heart and arteries including heart attack and stroke. That's because, quite literally, I had to fight heart disease to save my own life. My motivation back in 1984 was to survive to raise my two children. The risk of dying of a repeat bypass surgery, I was told, was five to six times as great as the first operation, owing to a variety of possible complications. The day I heard those statistics from the surgeon scheduled to do that second bypass was my moment of epiphany.

I swore that, if I survived, I would devote all my capabilities as a trained medical journalist to learning all I could about heart disease in general and cholesterol in particular. That's because I had already given up smoking cigarettes and my blood pressure was considered normal, and because then in 1984 more and more medical authorities were coming to the conclusion that cholesterol was a major risk factor. It was in 1987 that the US National Institutes of Health, together with the nation's medical organisations, formed the National Cholesterol Education Program to urge all men and women to get their cholesterol levels checked and, if raised, to get them down.

It was in that same year that I published my book *The 8-Week Cholesterol Cure*, detailing the programme I developed to get my own cholesterol levels down from a dangerously high 269 to 184 in just eight weeks without the use of prescription drugs. I'm the guy who put oat bran in the diet in the US and around the world. It was years later that the US Food and Drug Administration for the first time gave permission for a food to make a health claim, namely that oats, along with a low-fat diet, could help prevent heart disease.

Since then I've devoted my life to studying heart disease and the latest developments on how to prevent it. I've applied those principles to my own heart-healthy regimen and have shared them with my readers by way of my quarterly publication *The Diet-Heart Newsletter* and a number of books including a total rewrite of the original, *The New 8-Week Cholesterol Cure*.

I've achieved my goal of sticking around long enough to raise my children, who have graduated from college and are now completely on their own. But I've set the pole higher. I want to be around to play with my grandchildren some day. And I'm happy to report that my doctors, having regularly tested my heart, think I'll be able to do just that. Not to brag, but rather to inspire, I'm in great health, with a completely unlimited lifestyle.

But I continue to modify and improve my own regimen as I learn new approaches. And that's why the newest, seventh edition of guidelines issued by the Joint National Committee (JNC-7) on blood pressure and hypertension in the USA in 2003 really caught my attention. For years, I'd thought that my own blood pressure was perfectly fine, and so did the doctors who examined and tested me. The new guidelines, however, labelled me as pre-hypertensive. At first, I dismissed the stricter limits as being overly cautious. Actually, a lot of doctors reacted the same way. After all, my numbers, typically around 125/78 mmHG, seldom more than 130/80 mmHG, had been considered normal and no doctors had ever talked about a need to lower it.

Then I started to read more about the subject. The data were compelling and overwhelming. The lower one's blood pressure, the lower the risk of cardiovascular disease. And blood pressure measurements previously considered normal actually predicted future risk.

Coincidentally, at the same time the medical community was coming to the conclusion that the lower one's cholesterol the better. I had accepted that idea years before, and did everything I could to keep my levels of 'bad' LDL cholesterol as low as possible and counts of 'good' HDL cholesterol as high as possible. Why shouldn't I view blood pressure with the same aggressive stance?

As with cholesterol control, however, I did not want to take prescription drugs. The JNC-7 guidelines called for lifestyle modifications including increased exercise and weight control before resorting to those drugs for pre-hypertensive patients. But I was already very physically active and at a healthy weight. So I started looking for natural, non-prescription approaches, just as I had done nearly two decades earlier for cholesterol control. I'll explain that term 'pre-hypertension' and compare and contrast US and UK guidelines in greater detail in the first chapter.

While I had studied blood pressure and hypertension rather extensively during my postgraduate physiology training, my first real encounter on a personal level came during a game of golf with my father in 1967. It seemed that he needed to find a tree or a bush on practically every other hole to urinate. It turned out that Dad had been prescribed a drug called a diuretic to control his hypertension, which was extremely severe.

Not much was known about how to prevent heart attacks and strokes back in those days, but high blood pressure was already considered a major culprit. Unfortunately, doctors knew even less about how to control hypertension other than with the first anti-hypertensive drugs. And, as is still the case today, those drugs had a long list of side effects, not least of which was the nuisance my father experienced with the need for frequent urination and fatigue. Many, if not most, men had greatly diminished sex drive, too.

Combine Dad's hypertension, high cholesterol levels, the major stress he experienced at the time and the lack of effective countermeasures, and we lost my beloved father in 1969 at the age of just 57. He and I were very close, and I miss him to this day and always will. Dad would have made a wonderful grandad, but never got to meet his grandchildren and bounce them on his knee.

As I said earlier, I'm one of the lucky ones who survived my fight with heart disease. For many, the first symptom is a fatal heart attack. And I intend to stay lucky. But, as someone once said, the harder one works at something, the luckier one gets. And so it was that in 2003 I turned my attention to getting my own blood pressure lower. I succeeded in doing just that, and now I want to share my findings.

For millions of men and women, following the simple steps I'll describe can keep blood pressure from rising during the coming years. For millions more, this complete programme of lifestyle modification and supplementation with completely safe and harmless substances can bring mild to moderate hypertension under control. And for those whose hypertension is so severe that it definitely requires prescription medications, the programme can keep doses as low as possible, thereby limiting side effects and adverse reactions.

As the old song goes, 'Little things mean a lot'. Sure, we'll talk about increasing levels of physical activity, controlling weight, stopping smoking and coping with stress and depression. But some simple supplements including a special formulation of grape seed extract, tomato extract, co-enzyme Q10 and folic acid can each provide a little reduction in blood pressure. Putting them into a complete programme gives 'a lot of bang for the buck'. And I've learned little tricks such as taking my daily aspirin tablet at night rather than in the morning, along with a tiny dose of melatonin, that help to keep BP down even lower during hours of sleep.

Then there's an amino acid, one of the building blocks of protein available in supplement form, one of my 'Secret Weapons' against blood pressure. That amino acid, l-arginine, is the precursor of a gas produced by the lining of the arteries to keep those arteries nice and elastic and flexible (see page 219). That, in turn, leads to lowered blood pressure since healthy arteries are more capable of dealing with increased blood flow throughout the day but especially during times of physical or mental stress.

Until recently, however, findings in research laboratories around the world didn't have a practical application since the l-arginine had to be continuously available in the blood stream. The typical arginine supplement taken orally, rather than by infusion directly into a vein in a hospital, brings levels up quickly but just as quickly disappears. The breakthrough moment came with the development of a sustained-release (SR) formulation that keeps arginine at an optimal level in the blood throughout the day and night.

University of Texas research shows that taking SR arginine allows for greater blood supply to the heart muscle. And subjects in the studies experienced lower blood pressures, especially if those numbers were high to begin with.

With all due respect for doctors, and I give them full credit for helping to keep me alive, they're often too quick to reach for the prescription pad without giving safer and more acceptable alternatives a fair chance. Part of it comes through past experience in finding that simply telling patients to lose weight and consume less salt doesn't do much to bring blood pressure down.

Furthermore, no one should really expect doctors to keep up with every new little discovery, especially when it comes to supplements. Tell the average GP that a few capsules of grape seed extract or an amino acid will significantly lower blood pressure, and he or she will likely roll his or her eyes.

I remember very well when my book introduced oat bran to the world as a way to lower cholesterol levels. A lot of doctors throughout the medical community thought it was hype and hokum. The research was there, but in journals seldom read by practising doctors.

So don't be surprised if your doctor is more than a little sceptical when you say you want to try the programme detailed in this book before you resort to those prescription drugs. That said, hypertension can be so severe that one must bite the bullet and accept the fact that drugs can't be avoided. The end – saving your life – surely justifies the means. I've devoted a chapter to those pharmaceutical agents to help you to understand how they work and why certain drugs are best for different individuals. Even then, however, following the programme in this book can and will allow you to keep the doses of those drugs, and thus their side effects, to a minimum.

Ironically, at least one aspect of blood pressure prevention and control remains controversial and, at the risk of sounding like a heretic, has been greatly exaggerated. That's salt and sodium in the diet. This deserves, and gets, a whole chapter in this book. But the essence of the truth is this: not everyone is salt sensitive and responds positively to salt restriction. And even those who *are* salt sensitive would have to follow restrictions so severe that the results will typically be negligible.

As with most matters, the salt issue isn't black and white but, rather, a shade of grey. Sodium, the 'offending' part of the salt molecule, sodium chloride, is just one of a group of chemical substances in the body called electrolytes. They also include calcium, magnesium and potassium. The body requires a balance of all the electrolytes. So, rather than merely cutting back on sodium, the trick is to consume more of the others. Research has shown very convincingly that doing so significantly improves blood pressure.

By the time you finish reading this book, you'll have a very good grasp of just what blood pressure and hypertension are. You'll learn that the ideal level is about 115/75. Those numbers reflect pressure measured in millimetres of mercury (mmHG) either in your GP's surgery or with a home unit. The top number, the systolic, is the pressure of major and minor arteries at the time the heart beats. The lower number, the diastolic, is a measurement of the pressure when the heart is at rest.

As one professor of anatomy told me, we're all as different on the inside as we are on the outside. So I've devoted a chapter to special considerations for men, women and children, and for different ages and races. And since diabetic individuals are at particular risk, I've paid extra attention to their needs.

Sure, I'm going to ask you to make some changes in your patterns of eating and physical activity. But I think you'll agree that the suggestions I make won't be radical or unreasonable. Almost no one is willing to change his or her life completely, so this will be more a matter of taking 'baby steps' to help get your pressure down to where it belongs and to protect against heart attack and stroke.

As usual, I've 'experimented' with myself and with my family and friends, especially with some of the dietary suggestions. One particular winner is getting into the habit of making fruit smoothies or shakes as a quick breakfast. Each smoothie contains four to five servings of fruit, enough to make a dietitian smile for the entire day. Try one and you'll be hooked. Another component of my daily programme is a relaxing cup of hot cocoa at bedtime.

It's important to note that none of the supplements that

are part of this programme have any potential for side effects or adverse reactions. And I've documented each and every suggestion with research studies published in the world's most prestigious medical journals. Both you and your doctor will be very happy with the results you can achieve with this complete programme of optimising your blood pressure.

Did the programme work for me? Absolutely! From previous readings at their highest of the high 130s/80s my numbers are now as low as 111/68.

In a nutshell, this book's programme will show you ways to attain a healthy weight, cope with stress, get the physical activity you need without having to go to the gym, enjoy a delicious diet that actually lowers blood pressure without deprivation, and use newly researched supplements that are often as effective as prescription drugs. The concepts are all solidly based on research carried out in the world's top medical centres and published in the most prestigious journals. And I've had doctors review what I've written to assure absolute accuracy. I've done my part. I've controlled my own blood pressure and now I'm sharing the information I've learned with you. Now it's up to you to do your part.

The foundation of this programme is spelled out in the first chapters, in which I explain what blood pressure is, how to measure it most accurately, and lifestyle modifications including coping with stress, weight control, dietary improvements, physical activity and so on. Whether you prefer the natural approach that I advocate or the use of prescription anti-hypertensive drugs for blood pressure control, that foundation is essential. But you'll find the really exciting and truly revolutionary breakthroughs in natural blood pressure control in Chapter 13, Little Things Mean a Lot, and Chapter 14, Secret Weapons Against the Silent Killer. You wouldn't be 'cheating' to jump right to those chapters. That way you can put some of those things to work for yourself immediately.

Got any doubts about whether it's all worth the effort?

Just think about everything you love in this life. Taking the pressure off your heart can add years of life and improve both the quality and quantity of those years. Yup, it's really worth it.

Recall the image of the crystal ball. You can, indeed, take a look into your future health by learning what your blood pressure and cholesterol numbers are like. And, if raised, you can take steps to get them under control. Really and truly, it's like stepping off a railway line if a train is bearing down on you. Your doctor can help, but to a large extent you hold your destiny in your own hands. I took steps to achieve heart health, and I know that you can too!

And after reading this book, I know you'll want to stay in touch with the latest developments in heart health in general and blood pressure control in particular. To do so please visit my website www.thehealthyheart.net. It's completely free, no subscription fee required.

Chapter 1
The Silent Killer

Blood pressure is rather like the weather. Everyone talks about it, but, in the case of blood pressure, not enough people do anything about it. It's often called the 'silent killer' because, for the most part, it has no symptoms. Headaches associated with blood pressure are relatively rare. We see hypertension mentioned over and over again as one of the major risk factors for heart attack and stroke. Every time we visit our GP's surgery we get our blood pressure tested. But the sad fact is that while literally millions of men and women have blood pressure levels that put them at risk, most don't get their numbers under control.

I think there are two reasons for that. First, most of us really don't understand blood pressure in a way that we can really appreciate its importance. Second, many people aren't willing to take drugs that carry a heavy load of side effects or to make what they perceive would be the major lifestyle sacrifices needed to eliminate a risk factor that doesn't appear to really bother them. In the next few pages, and in the balance of this book, you'll learn everything you need to know about blood pressure (BP) and you'll be delighted to find out that most people who have mild to moderately raised blood pressure levels don't have to make major changes in their lives or to take prescription drugs.

First of all, you already know more about BP than you realise. That's because you're very familiar with the plumbing in your own house. One of the great pleasures of life is taking a shower with water gushing powerfully over our bodies. That comes from having sufficient water pressure in our bathroom pipes. We also need good water pressure to wash the dishes and water the lawn and wash the car. Conversely, we all know the frustration of low water pressure. We might even have to call the plumber if the pressure falls too low. He or she'll use a little device to measure the pressure at different points in the house and garden and make suggestions as to how you can improve the situation. Maybe mineral deposits have clogged the plumbing. Once the problem or problems are fixed, you can have water pressure on demand.

Pretty easy to understand? I think we can all relate to that scenario. Well, it's really not so different from blood pressure. When we're young, our arteries – our internal pipes – are flexible and elastic and allow blood flow to be controlled without any problem. But as we age, and owing to other causes, our arteries stiffen and are unable to widen (dilate) and narrow (constrict) adequately as needed to provide our bodies with enough blood and oxygen. That explains 90 per cent of cases of hypertension, medically referred to as primary hypertension. In Afro-Caribbeans, an increase in blood output when the heart's ventricle pumps also plays an important role, as does their greater sensitivity to salt and sodium. Going back to the water pipe analogy, it's a gradual process we scarcely notice. Tragically, the first 'symptom' might be a heart attack or stroke. I've written this book to help eliminate such a tragic occurrence in your life.

So, enough about those water pipes. What about blood pressure? We'll start with the heart, which is essentially a marvellously designed chunk of muscle and chambers that pumps blood through an extensive network of arteries to every tissue in the body. Blood then returns to the heart through a parallel system of veins, where it collects in two chambers called the atria. Valves then permit that blood to enter the other two chambers, the ventricles. Blood leaving the heart has been oxygenated by the lungs and brings that oxygen to our muscles and other tissues. When blood returns, it is reoxygenated and gathers in the atria. Then the heart's left ventricle forcefully pumps oxygenated blood out through the aorta and on to the rest of the body's arteries.

Blood pressure is the force of our blood pushing against the walls of our arteries. As our hearts beat, typically 60 to 70 times a minute when we're sitting or lying down, blood is forced into and through the arteries. BP is highest when the heart beats, pumping that blood. That's the systolic pressure. Between beats, when the heart is at rest, BP falls. That's the diastolic pressure. BP is expressed as the systolic pressure over the diastolic pressure, as in 120 over 80, written as 120/80. We'll get into detail as to how blood pressure is tested and how those numbers are determined in the next chapter.

There are three known methods by which the body controls blood pressure. First, there are pressure receptors in various organs that can detect changes in BP and then adjust the pressure by altering both the force and speed of the heart's contractions, as well as the total resistance to pressure. Second, the kidney is responsible for long-term adjustment of BP through a system involving various chemical substances in the so-called renin-angiotensin system. Third, the steroid hormone aldosterone is released from the adrenal glands, which are located on top of the kidneys, in response to either high levels of potassium or angiotensin. This hormone then increases the excretion of potassium by the kidneys, while increasing sodium retention. For many readers, this information may be far more than they need, but I provide it here for those with some interest in the medical background.

But what happens when the arteries, an essential part of our cardiovascular systems, fail to perform optimally? Let's say that a woman finds herself under heavy emotional stress. A man goes out on an autumn day to sweep the leaves that have fallen. A fairly young guy decides to join in a kick-about game of football after too many years of sedentary lifestyle. In all three cases, the heart beats faster to pump out more blood than usual. But the arteries aren't up to the task, unable to convey that needed blood to the heart and the brain because those vessels can't dilate to accommodate the larger-than-usual blood volume. Pressure on the walls of the arteries increases, but the artery just can't open up enough. Additionally, some fatty plaque that has built up in the walls of the arteries may rupture, spilling its contents into the bloodstream, which precipitates the formation of a large blood clot. The result: heart attack or stroke. The aftermath of a stroke can be devastating for those who survive. While heart attacks and strokes most typically involve a number of factors, extreme hypertension, medically termed 'malignant', can alone be responsible.

Okay, okay, enough of the potentially tragic devastation of life. The good news is that most such heart attacks and strokes can be prevented by controlling – by 'curing' – the risk factors that cause them. The more we learn, the better the news gets. Based on data from the National Health and Nutrition Examination Survey in the United States, an ongoing decades-long evaluation, as many as three out of four cardiovascular 'events' could be prevented by optimal control of blood pressure and cholesterol. That conclusion came from studying the data from 1,921 people aged 30 to 74. Interestingly, that dramatic saving of life could be accomplished by bringing blood pressure down to levels most doctors would still believe to be too high, no more than 140/90. This book will show you how to get those numbers down much lower, improving your odds even more.

As early as 1957, the Metropolitan Life Insurance Company published a chart showing that as blood pressure levels rose, life expectancy fell. Conversely, the lower the levels, the longer the life. And who doesn't want a long, healthy life?

Hypertension – high blood pressure – has, for decades, been recognised as one of the 'Big Three' risk factors for cardiovascular disease, along with raised cholesterol levels and cigarette smoking. Because of what we now know, diabetes has been added to the list of major risk factors, one of the Big Four. Of course, genes and family medical history play a huge role. But those genetic traits simply predispose you to problems down the road. Eliminate the risk factors that convert the potential to the real, and the question of family history becomes virtually moot. When I began 'preaching' that mantra 20 years ago, many doctors said I was exaggerating or over-simplifying. The fact is that, as far back as 1978, actuarial tables that predict lifespan had pointed to death within ten years for a man of 35 with a family history, a long list of risk factors, and a heart attack and bypass surgery. That means that I should have been dead by the age of 43, sooner rather than later. But I guess I fooled them! Today the vast majority of doctors and medical authorities agree that cardiovascular diseases, and death from heart attacks and strokes, are largely preventable. You simply have to make the decision, as I did, to eliminate those risk factors. As virtually any doctor will tell you, the risk posed by hypertension can be completely eliminated.

Here's a very happy thought, something to help boost your commitment to good health in general and blood pressure control in particular. Several – not just one or two – trials have demonstrated without doubt that reductions in systolic blood pressure of as little as one to three points can decrease the relative risk of stroke by as much as 20 to 30 per cent. That's one heck of a return on your investment!

What is the impact in the United Kingdom and elsewhere?

Globally, the percentages of men and women whose blood pressure exceeds optimal limits and those who have blood pressure high enough to be defined as hypertension – 140/90 or more – continues to increase. In the UK today, six professional societies have joined together to promote a heart healthy population. They include the British Cardiac Society, the British Hypertension Society, Diabetes UK, Primary Care Cardiovascular Society and the Stroke Association. High blood pressure (hypertension) affects approximately 40 per cent of adults in England and Wales, and the National Health Service spends 15 per cent of its drugs budget on treatments for the condition.

According to statistics from the Heart Foundation in Australia, 28.6 per cent of the population has high blood pressure, that is more than 600,000 men and women. More than half of those are untreated – and possibly undiagnosed – and even more have not achieved adequate control. Such untreated individuals fall into definite categories: male, younger, not diabetic or obese, normal cholesterol, current smoker, excessive alcohol intake and insufficient physical activity. And they don't know they have a time-bomb ticking away in their hearts because they have no symptoms. The numbers are even more dramatic when one also considers those in what is now called the state of 'pre-hypertension', which we'll discuss shortly.

High blood pressure, the Heart Foundation says, causes the third greatest burden of disease in Australia – over 5 per cent of the total burden of disease and injury, second only to tobacco smoking and physical inactivity.

Statistics from the American Heart Association in the US in 2006 show that 65 million men and women have high blood pressure, defined as systolic pressure of 140 mmHG or more and/or a diastolic pressure of 90 mmHG or greater.

The good news is that mild and moderately raised blood pressure respond very well to lifestyle modifications and to the 'Secret Weapons' I describe in the programme in this book. Very few people will require the use of drugs, and even those who do will be able to limit the dosage they need – and thereby side effects and adverse reactions – by following this programme.

Hypertension risk factors – and what we can do about them

Family history certainly plays a large role in determining whether you will develop hypertension. But I prefer to think about that as a warning. If the barrier comes down and the lights come on at a railway crossing, you've got a pretty good idea that a train is on its way. The wise person wouldn't put himself or herself in harm's way by trying to race a car across the line. Just because your grandfather had hypertension and died from a stroke doesn't mean you can't take steps to avoid repeating that history.

Race definitely comes into play. High blood pressure is far more common in black people than in any other racial group – and hits at an earlier age. But we know that black people are far more sodium sensitive than white people and yet often consume a diet that is high in sodium, doubling the problem. The solution seems pretty obvious. Similarly, obesity and diabetes are more prevalent among these two groups. Rather than wringing one's hands in despair, the wise individual will take appropriate action.

High blood pressure is more common in young and middle-aged men than in women of similar ages. But the opposite is true as women hit 60 years of age and older. Testing, a simple and painless way to know if you're at risk, is available to everyone, regardless of sex.

And you can certainly take control of the other risk factors involved in the gradual progression of raised blood pressure and subsequent hypertension. Obesity plays a big part. The greater your body mass, the more blood needed to supply oxygen and nutrients to your muscles and other tissues. Obesity increases the number and length of blood vessels and therefore increases the resistance of blood that has to travel longer distances through those vessels. Increased resistance increases blood pressure. Moreover, fat cells themselves manufacture substances that adversely affect both heart and blood vessels.

Sedentary behaviour boosts your risk by 'deconditioning' the heart muscle – just as it does the other muscles in the body. Couch potatoes tend to have faster heart rates because their heart muscles aren't as efficient and have to work harder to pump blood. Moreover, physical activity is a vasodilator; that is to say, exercise of any sort dilates – widens – blood vessels. Combining inactivity with overweight multiplies the problem.

Sodium and salt intake remain controversial as risk factors for hypertension. While it's true that some individuals are particularly sensitive to sodium, whether from the saltcellar or the sodium-based ingredients in processed and fast foods, not everyone responds equally. And, as we'll see, sodium is but one of many minerals – or electrolytes – that affect blood pressure. Increasing intake of the others may be as important or more important as decreasing intake of sodium, other than for those who are proven to be sodium sensitive.

Alcohol definitely affects blood pressure. But this is as much a grey area as a black and white issue. Excessive consumption can raise BP while moderate drinking may actually help keep it in control.

Stress is another highly controversial subject in the medical research community, though doctors in clinical practice see the effects in their patients regularly. Stress increases production of harmful substances, increases heart rate and blood requirements, and over time can raise blood pressure and precipitate a heart attack and stroke. Again, there are many effective, proven methods to help cope with stress.

Symptoms of high blood pressure or hypertension

For the most part, hypertension is, indeed, a silent killer with no symptoms to tip you off that something might be wrong. An exception would be those who experience a dull headache, typically at the back of the head and usually in the morning. Bear in mind that such headaches are the exception rather than the rule.

Ordinary headaches, dizziness and nosebleeds are not symptoms, at least at the early stages of raised blood pressure. Those symptoms can occur, however, with severe hypertension. That said, even those with very high blood pressure don't normally have any symptoms.

Because blood pressure is influenced by a cascade sequence of chemical substances in the kidney, and because severely high blood pressure can damage the kidney, certain symptoms may occur in advanced disease states not directly due to blood pressure but, rather, to kidney damage. These include excessive perspiration, muscle cramps, weakness, frequent urination and rapid or irregular heartbeat.

Blood pressure classification

There has been considerable discussion, if not controversy, worldwide over the classification of raised blood pressure. This was precipitated in 2003 by the Joint National Committee on Blood Pressure and Hypertension (JNC), a branch of the National Institutes of Health in the US. Their seventh set of guidelines for classification and treatment (JNC-7) started what future medical historians might ultimately view as a revolutionary landmark in addressing the vital importance of blood pressure control at virtually all levels. Critics, however, both within and outside of the US, consider JNC-7 to be inflammatory and unnecessary. I'll discuss the nuances and let you judge for yourself, viewed from your vantage point as patient, doctor or both.

In the UK, current guidelines are virtually identical to those used in the US. There is just one difference, and that is the use of the term 'high normal' rather than 'pre-hypertension'. I'll explain fully.

In any case, here's the chart provided to Australian doctors from the Heart Foundation for use in diagnosing and treating patients aged 18 and older. It's from 'Hypertension Management Guide for Doctors 2004'.

Definitions and classification of blood pressure levels (mmHg)

Category	Systolic	Diastolic
Normal	less than 120	less than 80
High-Normal	120–139	80–89
Grade 1 (mild)	140–159	90–99
Grade 2 (moderate)	160–179	100–109
Grade 3 (severe)	more than 180	more than 110
Isolated systolic hypertension	more than 140	less than 90

By way of comparison, that classification chart is virtually identical to that used in the US until JNC-7 was issued. Here's the way the chart has been redrawn as of 2003.

Category	Systolic	Diastolic
Optimal	115 or less	75 or less
Normal	less than 120	less than 80
Pre-hypertension	120–139	80–89
Stage 1 hypertension	140–159	90–99
Stage 2 hypertension	more than 160	100 or more

Either the systolic (upper) or diastolic (lower) number needs to be raised to be placed into the appropriate category of pre-hypertension, stage 1 hypertension or stage 2 hypertension.

Why the big deal? What's the difference, you might well ask. As I'll detail shortly, risk of cardiovascular disease, heart attack, stroke and death rise linearly with blood pressure. The higher the level – anything over 120/80 – the greater the risk, especially when other risk factors are present at the same time, such as raised cholesterol levels, cigarette smoking and, especially, diabetes. The data are compelling. As you read through them shortly, you'll no doubt prefer to be at the low end of the risk spectrum. Doctors have sometimes been accused of not being aggressive enough in confronting and battling disease, especially degenerative disease that takes a long time to develop. Not any more!

But the biggest point of dissent was the introduction of the term 'pre-hypertension'. With some justification, critics feared that labelling patients as having 'pre-hypertension' rather than 'high-normal' blood pressure would make them fearful. Some were concerned that such a label on a medical record might influence medical insurance rates. And others worried that anti-hypertensive drugs might be prescribed excessively, even though the JNC-7 guidelines call for lifestyle modifications before prescribing drugs.

When I first read the JNC-7 guidelines, I sided with the critics. But the more I thought about it, the more I agreed that stricter guidelines were better. Interestingly, I had vehemently criticised US cholesterol guidelines for years, complaining to my readers that it was ridiculous to have two sets of guidelines, one for those without cardiovascular disease and another for those who had had a confirmed diagnosis or who had suffered a cardiovascular event of one sort or another. Wouldn't it be better to recommend that everyone get his or her LDL as low as possible and HDL as high as possible to *prevent* development of the disease or suffering of an event rather than waiting for that to happen?

And so it is with blood pressure. The lower we can get our numbers, the better off we will be now and in the future. All cardiologists and medical authorities agree that your goal should be 120/80 or, even better, down as low as 115/75 or lower. Guidelines of the Joint British Societies (JBS2) broadened the definition of risk. However, the UK guidelines still allow for higher levels, 160/100, prior to aggressive treatment.

Health authorities around the world have gradually begun to understand that the lower the level of blood pressure, the less risk there is of heart attack and stroke. Before one reaches a very high level, 160/100 or more, one can personally start taking steps to lower blood pressure.

But that doesn't mean you or I should turn into neurotics about our blood pressures, which the critics fear. Life is to be lived and enjoyed. And, happily, a lot of the things we can do to benefit our BP will make our lives even longer and more enjoyable!

The rationale for lower blood pressure

The data indicating that the higher the blood pressure, even within limits previously considered completely normal or high-normal, the greater the risk of cardiovascular disease, stroke, heart attack and death have been building up for several years. Those data have reached 'critical mass' and now virtually all doctors and medical authorities agree that the lower a person can bring his or her BP into an optimal zone of about 115/75 or even less, the better. And it now appears that, especially for those over 50, the systolic (top) number is most important. Even if the diastolic (bottom) number is quite normal, attention should be paid to getting the systolic pressure down. In fact, there is a condition termed 'isolated systolic hypertension' in which diastolic pressure is relatively normal but systolic pressure is raised. Doctors treat that condition aggressively.

In a study at the University of North Carolina involving about 9,000 men and women over a period of 11.6 years, the rate of cardiovascular disease increased significantly as blood pressure levels increased. Compared with patients with optimal BP levels, those with high-normal measurements had two and a half times the risk of developing cardiovascular disease. And that statistic took into consideration other factors involved in the disease. Most of the risk was in the form of stroke. And risk was greatest in black people, diabetics, overweight and obese individuals, and those with high levels of LDL cholesterol.

Researchers concluded that the 'pre-hypertension population is large' and that efforts to lower BP into optimal levels 'have the potential to make a significant impact'.

Subsequent investigations have proved that to be absolutely true. In a recently published study, nearly 9,000 middle-aged adults with blood pressure previously considered to be normal or high-normal were divided up into three groups and monitored for an average of 12 years. Blood pressures in the three groups were

- lower than 120/80
- 120–129/80–84
- 130–139/85–89

Compared to the group with the lowest blood pressure, the second and third groups had 70 per cent and 144 per cent greater risk, respectively, for coronary heart disease.

Moreover, high-normal BP often quickly progresses to frank (confirmed) hypertension within a period of four years or less. The older one is, the greater that risk. In a study at Boston University, nearly half of all adults aged 65 or older who had high-normal BP went on to develop hypertension during that time. And the likelihood of developing hyper-tension was increased an additional 20 to 30 per cent for those who gained an extra 5 per cent of body weight. Results were similar between men and women. Researchers concluded that high-normal blood pressure is more similar to hypertension than it is to normal BP. In other words, there is a continuum.

Here's another sobering statistic from the US JNC-7 report. The higher the BP, the greater the risk. For individuals aged 40 to 70 years, each increment of 20mmHg in systolic BP or 10mmHg in diastolic BP *doubles* the risk of cardiovascular disease across the entire blood pressure range from 115/75 to 185/115. Let's put that into some specifics. Let's say your systolic BP increases from 115 to 135 over a period of time. Your risk has been doubled. Over the coming years, if the systolic pressure goes up by another 20mm to 155, your risk is doubled again. It's a very slippery slope! But the good news is that the opposite also applies. There is a continuous benefit as blood pressure levels fall closer and closer to that optimal level of 115/75. That should be everyone's target, the holy grail of heart health.

And we already know the benefits that can be derived from lowering levels of what is now called pre-hypertension to more optimal counts. Results of the study known as TROPHY (TRial Of Preventing Hypertension) were presented at the March 2006 meeting of the American College of Cardiology. The mean age of patients with pre-hypertension was 48.5 years; half were treated and the other half were not. At the end of the two-year trial, treatment was shown to reduce the risk of progression to hypertension by 66 per cent.

In the TROPHY study, treated patients received the anti-hypertensive drug candesartan. But success can be achieved by lifestyle changes alone, as proved by a project funded by the National Heart, Lung and Blood Institute of Health. Lifestyle changes that protected the subjects in that study from progressing from pre-hypertension to hypertension included weight loss, physical activity, moderation of alcohol consumption and a diet rich in fruits, vegetables and wholegrain cereals. In fact, an editorial accompanying the report published in the *New England Journal of Medicine* questioned the use of potent pharmacologic agents and suggested aggressive lifestyle modification as the superior approach.

British and other international readers might well comment, 'Okay, that's the American point of view. But it doesn't necessarily apply to us in other countries.' Sorry, but that's just not true. It would get boring, but I could cite study after study from countries around the world including Australia, Sweden, Italy, Germany, Finland, and, yes, the United Kingdom, coming to the same inevitable conclusion: if you want to protect yourself from cardiovascular disease, stroke, heart attack, heart failure and kidney disease, get your blood pressure down to that optimal 115/75 level – or at least as close as possible.

Chapter 2
Testing Your Pressure

To get the best performance and the longest life out of the tyres on your car, you need to maintain optimal air pressure. And to find out if your tyres are at the optimal pressure, you do a simple test, or have the garage do so. The same applies to the pressure on your heart and in your arteries. The first step is to have a simple, painless check-up carried out at your GP's surgery or health clinic.

Most men and women have had their blood pressure measured at one time or another. But, bearing in mind that many individuals have either pressures above optimal levels or indisputable hypertension without knowing it, if you haven't had a test lately, call your doctor's surgery and make an appointment. While you're there, it would be a good idea to have your cholesterol levels checked as well. Raised cholesterol levels are not only a major risk factor for heart attack and stroke in and of themselves, but also predispose a person to developing hypertension.

Traditionally, to test blood pressure, the GP or practice nurse inflated a cuff placed around the upper arm. He or she then listened for specific sounds through a stethoscope placed at the crook of the elbow as the cuff is gradually deflated. The first of those sounds signals the time the heart beats. The fifth and final sound notes the heart at rest between beats. The pressure at the time of those two sounds is noted in a column of mercury similar to a thermometer on a device called a sphygmomanometer, frequently mounted on the wall. The first, beating, pressure is termed systolic (the upper number, as in 120/80) and the second is the diastolic. Both are measured in millimetres of mercury (mmHg).

More commonly the GP's surgery or health clinic now uses a digital apparatus to test blood pressure, reducing the environmental impact of mercury. But the mercury sphygmomanometer is still considered the 'gold standard' and is used to calibrate the accuracy of other devices.

Many things affect blood pressure, and so it's best to have at least two and preferably three measurements done while there. To make a diagnosis of hypertension, rather than just somewhat raised levels, the doctor should test blood pressures during three separate visits.

Here are a few things you can do to make sure your test is as accurate as possible. Get a good night's sleep the night before your visit. Wear a shirt or blouse that can be easily rolled up the arm so that the cuff can be placed on bare skin. Sit with both feet on the floor. Ideally, relax for a few minutes before the test by taking a few deep breaths and thinking happy thoughts. If you're seeing the GP for some other reason, ask to have your pressure measured at the end, rather than the start, of your appointment.

Smoking and drinking caffeinated drinks can raise blood pressure for two or more hours. Conversely, an older person's pressure might be lower immediately after eating. It may be higher in the morning than in the afternoon or evening. Talking tends to make pressure go up, so it's best to remain silent during the test.

It's natural to experience a certain amount of anxiety before any test, and that might make the pressure go higher. So it's a good idea to have more than one measurement during your visit. Wait a few minutes after the first measurement, then have the test repeated, ideally a couple of times.

White coat, labile and masked hypertension

A lot of people, including myself, naturally feel slightly anxious when visiting the doctor. As a result, blood pressure (BP) may well be higher in that setting than when at home. Such increases are called 'white coat hypertension'. Often pressure will go down during the course of the visit, but not always. For this reason, home monitoring is getting more and more popular with patients and doctors. We'll get into testing yourself in more detail later.

Researchers in Japan investigated white coat hypertension (WCH) in 128 subjects. At home, their BP on average was 135/85 mmHG. In a clinical setting it rose to 140/90 mmHG. Many men and women experience even greater differences.

Until recently, medical authorities considered WCH to be benign. But the Japanese investigators wondered whether WCH might signal the future development of actual hypertension. Over a period of eight years, they compared patients with WCH with those whose blood pressure was normal in a clinical setting. Nearly twice as many WCH patients went on to develop hypertension as those with normal pressure. Risk of future hypertension was greater for men and for older and/or overweight individuals.

There are no known biochemical, physiological or personality predictors of WCH. That means neither you nor your doctor can tell whether you're one of at least 10 per cent of the population whose BP will be higher in the doctor's surgery than at home.

Interestingly, even those who are being treated for hypertension and whose BP is controlled by drugs can experience WCH. That was proved to be the case by medical investigators in Greece, who compared the responses of hypertensive patients with those of subjects with normal blood pressure. They suggested monitoring outside a clinical setting.

Blood pressure similarly rises with anxiety and stress during everyday life. That's a natural and usually harmless phenomenon. You're driving along the road, let's say, and a child runs out into the street and you slam on the brakes. BP goes up as a normal response. But it's also normal for the BP to return to stress-free levels after a few minutes.

Some individuals, however, have a condition called 'labile hypertension' in which BP stays up longer than it should. And those men and women are likely to experience increases in BP more frequently than others, responding more dramatically to the stress and anxiety that everyone has to some degree or another.

As with WCH, labile hypertension (LH) wasn't considered dangerous in the past. But it now sends a signal to doctors that the person is more likely than others to develop full-blown hypertension. While it's true that there are no symptoms of hypertension or high blood pressure, we all know when we're angry, frightened or would like to shoot someone. Those emotional states raise blood pressure. The question is how long does that pressure stay up? And the two ways of answering that question are home monitoring and ambulatory BP monitoring (ABPM). The latter involves wearing a device that continuously records BP through a 24-hour period. More about home and ambulatory monitoring later.

Lastly, we have individuals whose BP appears normal when in the doctor's surgery, but goes up outside the clinical setting. Such persons suffer from 'masked hypertension'. They are more likely to be male, young and have higher than normal heart rates, according to Israeli researchers. They suggest that masked hypertension (MH) may be caused, at least in some cases, by a high level of physical activity during the day. In the Israeli study, 11 per cent of subjects exhibited MH.

As with WCH and LH, MH is best revealed by monitoring BP either with occasional home monitoring or by wearing an ambulatory device provided by a doctor who, for whatever reason, suspects MH. MH is also known in the medical community as 'reverse white coat hypertension' and 'white coat normotension'. This is particularly insidious since such patients tend to be at even greater risk than those with more commonly detected hypertension.

Factors affecting blood pressure readings

Levels of blood pressure vary significantly throughout the day and night. The lowest pressure occurs during sleep. Conversely, virtually everyone has, to some degree or other, what is termed a 'morning surge' in BP.

Doctors have noted this tendency for many years, but the definitive study was carried out in 2003. Investigators from the US and Japan collaborated in the work, which determined that significant morning surges in BP present a major risk of stroke for elderly patients with hypertension. Previous work established a similar risk for people rising from an afternoon siesta. It's scary to think that taking a nap can actually be hazardous to one's health!

Morning surge is now medically defined as the difference in systolic BP during the first two hours after waking and rising minus the lowest level of systolic BP recorded during the day or, ideally, during sleep. The greater the difference, the higher the risk of stroke. In the 2003 study, those at highest risk had a whopping difference averaging 55mgHg.

Please note that risk of stroke was increased for elderly patients with established hypertension, *not* those with normal or minimally raised BP. Older hypertensive individuals, however, should be aware of this risk, and should determine whether they experience morning surge by carrying out either home or ambulatory monitoring.

Even the weather affects blood pressure. Daytime BP tends to be lower during the hot days of summer than during cold weather. That's true regardless of age. But elderly men and women with hypertension have higher BP at night when the weather is hot. Such individuals typically are treated with anti-hypertensive drugs to control their BP, and they and their doctors should be aware that just because BP might be measured as being lower in the summer days, their medication dosage should not be reduced.

Home and ambulatory blood pressure monitoring

Technology has taken great strides forward during the past decade or so. Most people today have access to a computer and many use one every day. Giant TV screens dominate family rooms, turning them into home theatres with DVD players. Mobile phones are everywhere, linking friends, family, and business people and professionals wherever they go.

Ten years ago, doctors scoffed at the idea of measuring and monitoring blood pressure at home rather than in the surgery. Today, many doctors, at least those 'in the know', recognise that modern home BP monitors are as good or perhaps even better, than clinical testing. That trend is worldwide.

Late in 2004, the American Heart Association advocated home monitoring in its revised guidelines for blood pressure measurements, published in the February 2005 issue of the journal *Hypertension*. The lead author of that report, Dr Thomas Pickering, of Columbia University, in New York, said, 'We've found that blood pressure measurements taken by doctors in their offices may actually be unreliable in many patients. For that reason, there is wider acceptance of blood pressure readings taken by patients in their homes, and of ambulatory blood pressure monitoring.'

Greek medical researchers found that home monitoring is actually superior to both clinical testing and ambulatory monitoring. They systematically tested and compared the three methods over a three-month period in 133 patients. The team determined that home monitoring produced the most accurate measurements. They wrote that such monitoring would lead to better success with prescription drugs to lower blood pressure, but that also applies, of course, to natural, non-prescription techniques of maintaining normal blood pressure and lowering raised levels.

Not only were the early home monitors inaccurate but they were also expensive. Today they are both accurate and inexpensive. They're a great investment in cardiovascular health for you and the entire family. Even children. Authorities advocate blood pressure testing for those aged at least 18 years old. And, if there's a family history of heart disease, hypertension and stroke, it's a good idea to start as young as 13. By the way, that also applies to testing for cholesterol levels. Because of my own battle with heart disease and my family history, I made a heart-healthy lifestyle a family affair well before my children entered their teens.

You'll find many brands in the marketplace. Omron makes excellent, reliable devices approved by the British Hypertensive Society, which is internationally recognised for evaluating monitors. I personally use the Omron HEM-737 Intellisense. Choose the type that employs a cuff wrapped around the upper arm. They are more accurate than wrist models. Be sure to select one with the proper size cuff for your body. Cuffs that are too large or too small reduce accuracy.

Even though the home monitoring devices are extremely easy to use, technique is important to assure accurate BP measurements. It's best to sit at a table or desk, wrap the cuff around the arm, as directed in the instructions, and relax for a couple of minutes before inflating the cuff. Keep both feet on the floor and try to remain still, since movement can affect the reading. Your arm and cuff should be at the same height as your heart. Hit the start button and note your BP. Many machines also measure heart rate. Wait a couple more minutes and repeat the procedure. You'll probably find that the first measurement is higher.

To establish what doctors call a 'baseline', keep a chart of your BP measurements at various times of the day. Jot down a few notes. Was it a hot day? Were you under a lot of stress?

Did you have a lot of coffee to drink that day? An alcoholic beverage? Do that for a week. Then periodically retest your BP. If it is raised and you begin to follow the suggestions in this book, you'll be pleased to see improvements in the coming weeks and months!

You'll want to share your data with your doctor. And it's a good idea to have your machine calibrated in his or her surgery, comparing the measurements you get on your home device with a mercury-based sphygmomanometer in a clinical setting.

What about the ambulatory BP monitoring (ABPM) I referred to? This employs an apparatus provided by the doctor and gives a 24-hour record of blood pressure levels, with readings taken at 15- to 30-minute intervals throughout the day and night. ABPM is used for patients with white coat hypertension, to determine whether morning surges are occurring, to measure BP during sleep, and to learn how well anti-hypertensive drugs are working. Typically, ABPM is prescribed for patients with severe hypertension, especially for the elderly. ABPM is becoming more popular among hypertension experts as being the most definitive method to truly determine a patient's risk. ABPM allows a doctor to determine the average BP throughout the day, a more informative measurement than a few tests at the surgery. For most individuals, however, home monitoring devices are more than adequate.

Classification of blood pressure for adults aged 18 and over

Classification	Systolic BP	Diastolic BP
Normal	less than 120	less than 80
Pre-hypertension	120–139	80–90
Stage 1 Hypertension	140–159	90–99
Stage 2 Hypertension	more than 160	more than 100

Chapter 3

Special Considerations for Special People

Raised blood pressure and hypertension know no ethnic or gender boundaries, afflicting men and women of all races all over the world. But every individual has special needs that must be taken into consideration.

Blood pressure and children

Cardiovascular disease in general and hypertension in particular begin in childhood. Studies indicate that children with raised blood pressure levels are more prone to develop hypertension later on, even as early as young adulthood. The percentages of youngsters with higher than normal blood pressure are increasing over time, perhaps owing to more sedentary behaviour and overweight. One estimate is that 30 per cent of all overweight children have raised BP. Doctors are now seeing children as young as five years with higher than normal blood pressure.

Not surprisingly, normal blood pressure for children is lower than that for adults and gradually increases over the years. On average, systolic pressure will increase by 0.44mm Hg annually for children aged between eight and 12 years old and by 2.90 mmHG between the ages of 13 and 17 years. Diastolic BP also rises gradually, by 0.33 mmHG from the age of eight to 12 years and by 1.81 from 13 to 17 years. Here's a little chart to show typical BP readings for youngsters between eight and 17.

Age	Blood Pressure in mmHg (millimetres of mercury)
8	100/57
9	103/60
10	102/62
11	107/59
12	101/59
13	104/59
14	109/61
15	110/62
16	111/66
17	117/66

Both blood pressure and cholesterol levels should be checked by the paediatrician or GP early in life, especially in those families with a history of cardiovascular disease and premature heart attack and stroke. For reasons I personally cannot comprehend, there has been some controversy about doing so. It seems logical to me that a parent would want to know whether a son or daughter has a greater than average potential to develop that disease later in life and to pay particular attention to encouraging a heart healthy lifestyle in the entire family, complete with a heart-smart diet and plenty of physical activity. What parent would *not* want to give his or her child a future free of heart disease?

Good habits can be encouraged early in life and developed as easily as bad habits. My son Ross was six years old and Jenny was just three when I had my second bypass surgery. I did not want them to grow up to face the suffering I had undergone. A child's lifestyle is entirely dependent, especially very early in life, upon his or her parents. If fruit slices replace potato crisps, kids will eat those healthier foods. If playing actively in the garden and park, with the whole family involved and perhaps the children of neighbours as well, becomes the norm, less time will be spent in sedentary behaviour. We encourage our children to study hard at school and do their homework. Why not be as interactive with their health as well?

If the paediatrician or GP doesn't automatically test for blood pressure during surgery visits, ask him or her to do so. Proper cuff size is critical to get accurate readings. One size does not fit all. A diagnosis of hypertension cannot be properly made at just one visit. Readings must be high on three separate occasions at least one week apart. One estimate I read indicated that only about 10 per cent of hypertensive children are diagnosed. That means that 90 per cent are left to continue developing cardiovascular disease. To me that's unforgivable.

While being overweight plays the biggest part in raised blood pressure in childhood, other factors also enter the picture. Certainly the doctor will check for underlying disorders that can influence BP. And since sleep disorders can affect blood pressure, be certain to mention any sleeping problems your child might be having. Smoking habits also play a role.

Swedish research shows that boys born prematurely have a significantly greater risk of developing hypertension in later life. Investigators studied more than 300,000 males who had been born between 1973 and 1981 and who were conscripted into military service between 1993 and 2001. Blood pressure readings of those young men who had been born prematurely were proportionately raised in a linear fashion depending on just how premature they were. Those born before 29 weeks had almost twice the risk of high blood pressure; those born moderately pre-term, from 33 to 36 weeks, had a 24 per cent greater risk. The researchers recommend that children born prematurely have their blood pressure tested. While this study involved only young men, and the conclusions cannot be extrapolated to young women, it would appear wise to test all children born prematurely.

Although hypertension is most typically 'silent' in adults, causing no symptoms, that's not always true for children. More than half of children with untreated raised blood pressure experience frequent headaches, sleeping difficulties, daytime tiredness and chest or other pains.

For most children with raised blood pressure, treatment begins and ends with attaining a healthy weight and becoming more physically active. Those with other underlying causes of hypertension should be properly treated. Occasionally a child's hypertension will be severe enough for the doctor to consider prescribing a drug. Ultimately that may be unavoidable. But why not attempt to lower blood pressure with one or more of the natural, harmless supplements I discuss in Chapter 14? There's nothing to lose and, potentially, everything to gain.

Blood pressure and black people

Afro-Caribbeans have one of the highest rates of hypertension in the world. Compared with white people, black people are far more likely to have high blood pressure, to be overweight or obese, to live sedentary lifestyles and engage in less physical activity, to have diabetes and to smoke cigarettes. That's a formula for disaster. Hypertension is the single largest factor for cardiovascular disease, stroke, kidney disease and heart failure in Afro-Caribbeans. Similar combinations of traits can be found in other populations, such as Native Americans, who also have higher incidence of hypertension. Ironically, in South Africa white men have a higher prevalence of hypertension than black men, though the situation is reversed in women there.

The correlation between race and hypertension goes beyond medical and/or physiological explanations. It appears that racism itself has been shown to increase blood pressure in black communities. That racism, according to researchers at Duke University, in North Carolina, doesn't even have to be overt; it can exert its influence just by being perceived. Doctors there measured 24-hour ambulatory blood pressure, with monitors attached to subjects' bodies measuring BP on a continuous basis throughout the day. Participants also filled out a report detailing episodes of racism and resultant anger. But in order to live in a racist environment, those black persons had to repress their anger.

The major finding was that the differential between sleeping and waking blood pressure was less than average and certainly less than desirable. The greater the difference between night and day BP the better. Psychologically, African-Americans were inhibiting their anger throughout the night in their subconscious thoughts, thus keeping blood pressure levels up.

The solution to the problem may well be more social than medical. In a project based at Johns Hopkins Medical Center, in Baltimore, Maryland, 309 urban African-Americans participated in a programme including job referrals, career training and housing assistance. At the end of a three-year period, the proportion of men who took part in the programme had significantly better control of their hypertension than those who did not participate.

Whether a reflection of the culture or of the pressures endured by lower socio-economic groups, the use of illegal drugs, cigarette smoking, alcohol abuse and poor dietary choices rich in saturated fats and sodium prevails in poor African-American communities. One also finds a more defeatist attitude that would lead to rejection of suggestions for self-help health improvement.

In the UK, dietary concerns are critical among Afro-Caribbeans. Culturally ingrained eating habits are cherished or at least greatly enjoyed. Dishes are traditionally extremely high in salt. At the same time, black people tend to be sodium sensitive. It's a matter of adding fuel to the fire. As such, the first drug of choice in this group most typically will be a diuretic to eliminate both stored fluids and sodium. Replacement of simultaneously lost potassium is essential, ideally by increasing potassium-rich foods and by encouraging use of salt replacement products that substitute potassium chloride for sodium chloride.

While there is no way scientifically to authenticate the following explanation of sodium sensitivity and hypertension in African-Americans, the logic is intriguing. When black Africans were loaded onto ships bound for America for the slave trade, conditions were deplorable. Slaves were kept in the bowels of the ships where temperatures soared. Drinking water was insufficient, and dehydration led to numerous deaths. It has been speculated that those slaves with a genetic trait for retaining salt and water were able to survive. And it is the genes of those surviving slaves that have been passed on through the generations in African-Americans who are descendants of those poor souls.

Women, hypertension and heart disease

Historically, doctors viewed heart disease as virtually the exclusive purview of men. Women with identical symptoms would often be diagnosed with something other than the heart disease that was, in fact, killing them. For decades, the bulk of the money spent on cardiovascular disease research was earmarked for studies involving men. Women were ignored. At best, an afterthought might be added to an article printed in a medical journal to the effect that the findings probably pertained to women as well as to men. In hindsight, that was not always true.

The fact remains that cardiovascular disease is the number one killer of both men and women. It is an equal opportunity agent of death. Yet despite years of efforts to educate women, surveys continue to show that females fear breast and ovarian cancers far more than they fear heart disease. One woman in eight will die of breast cancer; one in two will succumb to heart disease, dying of heart attack or stroke.

On levels beyond the obvious, women are very different from men. Their symptoms of a heart attack or angina pains will not be a dramatic crushing chest pain, or pain radiating from the left shoulder down the arm, or feelings of indigestion or tightening sensation in the jaw. Rather they might suffer a persistent and unexplained fatigue, feelings of lethargy and emotional disturbances. Doctors have until recently viewed such symptoms chauvinistically and have prescribed tranquillisers and sleeping aids.

Though improvements have been made, a report from the American Heart Association on 30 January 2006 indicated that:

- Women's chest pain is not taken as seriously as men's,
- Women with stable chest pains are less likely than men to be referred for diagnostic tests, receive heart bypass surgery, angioplasty (blood vessel surgery) or be prescribed heart medications,
- Women are more likely than men to be readmitted to the hospital after bypass surgery,
- Women are more likely to have a worse outcome than men after coronary bypass surgery.

The intrinsic nature of women to put the needs of others, their family and friends, ahead of their own prevents them from seeking medical help at the first signs of cardiovascular disease. And when women do visit their GP with such symptoms, doctors will still frequently either misdiagnose or dismiss them. Women have a higher rate of morbidity and mortality from heart attack, stroke, angioplasty and bypass surgery than men, most likely because their disease has progressed far more by the time it is diagnosed. And for black women, the statistics are far worse.

Hypertension takes a greater toll on women than on men. The risk of repeat heart attacks, strokes and other cardiovascular events in women increases as blood pressure rises. In a prospective study of more than 5,000 female health professionals with an average age of 62, for each ten-point increase in systolic blood pressure a woman's cardiovascular disease risk increased by 9 per cent. High blood pressure makes the heart work harder in order to pump blood throughout the body; that, in turn, causes the heart to enlarge and lose efficiency over time.

In the above study, carried out at Brigham and Women's Hospital, in Boston, through the National Institutes of Health, researchers found increased risk started at a systolic pressure of 130. In the range of 130 to 139, systolic BP risk was 28 per cent greater than in women with a BP between 120 and 129. This is one more demonstration of the importance of paying attention to – and lowering levels of – what is now termed 'pre-hypertension'. Lifestyle modifications, especially in conjunction with new supplements, can effectively reduce pre-hypertension without the need for prescription drugs for women as well as for men.

The importance of one of those lifestyle modifications, increased physical activity, was highlighted at the 2004 meeting of the American College of Cardiology. Fitness in women was shown to be the most important factor in assessing cardiac mortality risk. Every increase in fitness, measured on a treadmill, was associated with a 9 per cent decrease in all-cause mortality and a 13 per cent drop in cardiac mortality.

Here are some things for women to think about in terms of dealing with blood pressure and preventing or treating hypertension. Women have unique considerations.

Are you taking the pill? Researchers have determined that taking oral contraceptives is linked with higher blood pressure in some women, particularly if you're overweight. It's also a major consideration if you developed high blood pressure during pregnancy, have a family history of hypertension or have kidney dysfunction. Taking contraceptive pills and smoking cigarettes is a dangerous combination. If you're thinking about starting on the pill, have your doctor measure your BP and discuss these other conditions. If you're already taking the pill, have your BP monitored regularly, at home or at the doctor's surgery or well woman clinic.

Hypertension can develop rapidly during the third trimester of pregnancy. Untreated, it can pose a danger to both mother and child. So-called gestational hypertension commonly disappears after pregnancy, but not always. And if your blood pressure was raised prior to pregnancy, it's particularly important to monitor it on a regular basis.

Without making any moral judgements, it is a fact that women are more prone to gain weight as they age and are more likely to become obese. Both overweight and obesity greatly increase the risk of raised blood pressure and hypertension.

Blood pressure tends to rise as both women and men age. But the risk of developing hypertension increases significantly following menopause.

If a woman's mother had high blood pressure, her odds of developing the disease increases substantially. That's also true for diabetes – in women and men. If you have those diseases in your family history, forewarned should be forearmed.

Blood pressure and the elderly

Throughout the Western world, as well as in rapidly developing nations, the percentage of elderly men and women is increasing rapidly. Blood pressure rises in step with advancing age. Data from the internationally renowned Framingham study show that 27 per cent of those aged under 60 years have blood pressure readings higher than 140/90 and 20 per cent have definite hypertension with measurements of 160/100. That's pretty bad. But among those aged over 80 years, nearly 75 per cent are hypertensive (higher than 140/90) and 60 per cent are at 160/100 or higher. Only 7 per cent of the oldest group studied, those aged over 80, had normal blood pressure.

Unfortunately, the percentage of hypertensive elderly men and women being treated is lower than doctors would like to see. And, of those receiving treatment, the number achieving desired blood pressure goals is far from desirable.

Many doctors still believe that aggressively treating elderly patients is unproductive. They maintain that few are willing to go along with medical advice. And some have said to me in private conversations that they don't want to ask older men and women to change their lifestyles, giving up some of their favourite foods and exercising more than they've done in perhaps decades. After all, such doctors say, those men and women don't have that many years left anyway, and they may as well enjoy all their simple pleasures. What a pile of condescending crap!

It has been my distinct pleasure to work with a number of organisations of elderly men and women, doing presentations for church groups, hospitals, self-help groups and retirement communities. I started doing so shortly after my first book was published in 1987 and I've continued ever since. And I must say that of all audiences I address, none is more attentive and open to suggestions. I love it when I drive into retirement villages and see men and women in their sweatshirts and shorts briskly walking, arms pumping back and forth, along established paths.

I think those doctors I referred to above have lost perspective. Many elderly men and women are accurately described as 'Golden Agers'. They've worked hard all their lives, raised their children and are now enjoying their earthly rewards, in no particular hurry to seek their eternal ones. They love their grandchildren and enjoy spoiling them – in spite of the parents' disapproval. They look forward to their holidays, whether their financial circumstances allow for cruises on luxury ships in the Mediterranean or coach trips to the seaside. They take pleasure in gathering in community centres for bingo games, bridge tournaments or to hear a lecture from an author such as myself.

I leave those occasions with a huge smile on my face and feel that I've learned far more than I've taught. What I've learned is that no matter how old one gets, life is enjoyed more completely in good health and that health and vitality are worth working for. Those senior citizens are, indeed, willing to change their dietary habits – at least reasonably so. They'll engage in physical activity, especially when it can be fun, such as when gardening or walking with friends. And despite what many doctors believe, they're willing to take their medications – when they understand what those drugs do and how they work and what side effects, if any, might be expected. After all, they might say about such side effects, life has its trade offs.

Indeed, some of the side effects that might keep younger men and women from being compliant with their prescriptions become less troublesome for the elderly. If a pill causes one to become a bit tired in the middle of the day, it might be nice to take a nap! If a diuretic pill means more trips to the bathroom, that's okay too.

One of the potential added benefits of treating and controlling blood pressure in the elderly is a reduced risk of dementia. Investigators at the National Institute of Aging, in Bethesda, Maryland, have observed that the longer a person is treated for hypertension, that is to say, the sooner one begins to bring blood pressure under control, the lower the dementia risk becomes. These findings appear to dismiss previous concerns that lowering blood pressure might have a negative effect on cognitive function. Quite the opposite seems to be true. Compared with those who were never treated for hypertension, those in the study who had been treated for 12 years or more had 60 per cent less risk of dementia than those who had never been treated.

Ultimately your doctor will make the decision as to which drug or drugs might be best for you, at least to start with. And if you have a good relationship with him or her – as you should have, for heaven's sake – you can experiment until you find the winning combination.

Elderly individuals often have structural and functional damage to the aorta, the large artery leading from the heart, that causes increased stiffness and resultant increased blood pressure. Some studies have shown that calcium-channel blockers and diuretics are drug classes that are particularly useful in treating elderly hypertension. Perhaps that's because those drugs provide greater reductions in aortic pressures than other drugs such as beta-blockers. Other studies have come up with completely opposite conclusions. Work with your doctor as a doctor/patient team.

Read Chapter 15: Prescription Drugs: The Last Resort to Lowering Blood Pressure (see page 246). It'll be good for you to more completely understand how they work. You'll impress your doctor! And consider taking one or more of the supplements that can improve arterial health and reduce blood pressure naturally. Even if those supplements can't do the job on their own, and in elderly individuals they're less likely to do so, they can help reduce drug doses and improve the flexibility and elasticity of your arteries. That's a good thing.

As I come to the end of this chapter, I'm filled with a lot of thoughts. Memories of establishing heart-healthy habits in my children Ross and Jenny and happiness that both have carried those habits into young adulthood. Greater realisation of the problems of ethnic groups less fortunate than myself. The need to be supportive of my wife's special needs. And a flood of amazement that when I began doing those presentations at churches and hospitals and retirement villages I was considered a 'youngster' in my middle forties and now I'm approaching my own 'Golden Age'. But two things have definitely not changed: first, the burning desire to share helpful health information with others and, second, my own willingness to work as hard as ever to stay healthy myself, to forego those fatty but tasty dessert temptations and to exercise even when my muscles and bones complain in their inimitable achy language. Because life, indeed, is worth living to the fullest and the only way to do that is to stay as healthy as possible. The arthritis in my hands and the pain in my back from degenerative discs that come with being in my sixties won't hold me down!

Chapter 4

Diabetic Patients Must Learn Their ABCs

Most doctors I spoke to while researching this book said virtually the same thing: 'I consider every diabetic patient to be a heart patient.' That was confirmed by a 2002 survey carried out by the American Diabetes Association (ADA) and the American College of Cardiology (ACC). More than 90 per cent of doctors surveyed reported that men and women with diabetes are 'very' or 'extremely likely' to have a cardiovascular 'event'. Here in the UK, the National Institute for Health and Clinical Evidence (NICE) cites equal risk between patients with established heart disease and those diagnosed as having diabetes.

There's a good reason all those doctors feel that way. Fully 65 per cent of diabetic men and women will die from a heart attack or stroke. And yet diabetic patients are not sufficiently conscious of their risk. In another survey by ADA and ACC that same year, 68 per cent reported that they were not aware of their increased risk for heart disease and stroke. Indeed, those cardiovascular events such as heart attack strike diabetics more than twice as often as they do others.

A diagnosis of diabetes as an adult presents the same degree of risk as someone who has already had a heart attack. Cardiovascular complications happen at an earlier age and often result in premature death. Those with diabetes are five times more likely to suffer strokes and, after the first stroke, are two to four times more likely to have a second one.

While cardiovascular disease statistics seem to be improving for the general population, those gains are not shared by people with diabetes. Quite the contrary. Deaths from heart disease in women who have diabetes have increased by 23 per cent over the past 30 years while there has been a 27 per cent *decrease* in heart disease in women who don't have diabetes. Deaths for diabetic men have decreased by 13 per cent but men without diabetes have enjoyed a 36 per cent decrease. That's why it is absolutely essential that men and women with diabetes learn and practise their ABCs.

'A' stands for (haemoglobin, Hb) A1C or HbA_{1C}, otherwise known as glycated haemoglobin. This is a measurement of the effect that glucose (sugar) has on the protein (haemoglobin) in red blood cells over time and therefore indicates average glucose levels over the previous two- to three-month period. Have that test done at least twice a year. You'll want the results to be between 6.5 per cent and 7 per cent or less.

'B' represents blood pressure. We'll be discussing that in detail in this chapter. Your target should be less than 130/80mmHg, the definition of hypertension in diabetic individuals, as compared with 140/80 mmHG for those without the condition.

'C' stands for cholesterol, especially the 'bad' LDL cholesterol. Yours should be less than 3 mmol/l – in fact, as low as possible. You'll want to pay particular attention to Chapter 12: Eating Your Way out of the Pressure Cooker.

Hypertension: even more important in diabetes care

Hypertension is pervasive in those with diabetes. In the US, the Third National Health and Nutrition Survey (NHANES) found that:

- 71 per cent of all diabetic men and women had hypertension,
- 29 per cent of those were unaware that they had raised blood pressure and
- 43 per cent were untreated.

Even those being treated had a blood pressure of more than 140/90. And only 12 per cent on treatment had reached the goal of less than 130/80.

Diabetic men and women have an increased risk of developing pre-hypertension, if not full-blown hypertension. Pre-hypertension puts everyone, and especially those with diabetes, at greater risk of cardiovascular disease, and predicts that, if left uncontrolled, hypertension will follow. The risk of developing cardiovascular disease for diabetic individuals is 3.6 times as great as that for non-diabetic men and women with normal blood pressure. That's a huge difference in risk!

The good news, after all those dreadful statistics that I hated to report but felt I had to give you, is that diabetes in general and hypertension in particular can be controlled and complications and risks can be greatly reduced. The first step must be to make the commitment to yourself and to those you love and who love you.

A woman my wife Dawn worked with at the high school where they both taught was only in her early thirties but was obese. She actually requested that she be assigned no classes on the second floor because she was unable to walk up the stairs and there was no lift. She ate huge amounts of food and was completely sedentary. One day she told Dawn that her doctor diagnosed her as having diabetes. Her response was startling, saying that she expected to get the disease since her mother and grandmother both had it, but she hadn't expected to develop diabetes so soon. Yet even after that diagnosis the woman did nothing to lose weight or to become more active.

A friend of mine, who had already suffered a massive heart attack, was told by his doctor that if he did not control his diabetes, he was not only under great risk of a second attack but could expect lower limb amputations and kidney failure requiring dialysis. Surely, you would think, that got his attention. No, he has now lost a few toes and walks with a cane, undergoes dialysis that leaves him exhausted twice a week, and can no longer work.

Only you can make the commitment. I can only hope that since you're now reading this chapter and this book that you're open to suggestions that can not only save your life but also make your life a lot more enjoyable.

Controlling blood pressure and diabetes

In many ways, you have a two-for-the-price-of-one situation. The same lifestyle modifications detailed throughout this book will help to control both diabetes and high blood pressure. In fact, the guidelines for initial treatment of diabetics with a blood pressure reading of 130–139/80–89 call for a three-month trial of non-drug treatment prior to starting a patient on anti-hypertensive drugs.

Those modifications include weight loss, increased physical activity, smoking cessation, moderation of alcohol consumption and restricted sodium intake. All are detailed in this book. The ADA and ACC note in a publication for doctors that weight loss can reduce blood pressure, even without changing sodium, and that losing just 1kg results on average in a decrease of one point in blood pressure. How much weight should you lose? Only you can give an honest answer to that question. Whatever the number of kilos, each one lost can lower your BP by a point. That can be very significant. Increasing your physical activity to an average of 30 to 45 minutes per day most days of the week, with a brisk walk as an example, can further lower blood pressure.

The wonderful thing is that patients who lose a sufficient amount of weight and who become physically active may not only 'cure' their raised blood pressure but also diabetes itself. Daily measurements of glucose and periodic tests of HbA_{1C} can show a return to normal levels. The diagnosis of diabetes is tentatively made when blood glucose rises above 7mmol/l after the person has fasted for 8–14 hours. A definitive diagnosis is established by a reading of more than 7 per cent on the HbA_{1C} test. Conversely, when fasting blood glucose levels fall below 6mmol/l and HbA_{1C} is consistently less than 7 per cent, a person's diabetes is 'cured'. I use quotation marks here because once diabetes is established, the person must be vigilant on a lifelong basis to keep glucose and HbA_{1C} counts normal, lest diabetes return. But, for all practical purposes, your diabetes would be cured, without the quotation marks. And that means that the risk of cardiovascular disease and other complications of diabetes including potential kidney damage, blindness and amputations are greatly reduced. Isn't that worth working for?

Virtually all doctors feel that the vast majority of diabetic patients will require more than one drug, often as many as three, to control hypertension. Most doctors will begin with an ACE inhibitor (see Chapter 15) and add other drugs as needed. Those drugs, of course, come with a raft of potential side effects, so it would be well worth your while to do your level best to get your blood pressure down without needing them. Your doctor won't be disappointed. Trust me when I say that more doctors would give those lifestyle modifications more credence and be in less of a hurry to reach for the prescription pad if they felt that their patients would do their utmost to achieve the desired goals through weight loss, exercise, stress management and so on. Sadly, most patients do not, and doctors have come to expect that failure. Prove your doctor wrong!

While working hard to lose weight and increase physical activity, you'll also want to use the special 'Secret Weapons' in Chapter 14. All those supplements have been shown to increase levels of nitric oxide, as I explain, a gas that keeps arteries flexible, elastic, and capable of dilation to allow for increased blood flow as needed. They have all been shown to lower blood pressure. It's the pressure of blood flow against less flexible and elastic arteries that we call hypertension.

In reading that chapter, you'll want to pay particular attention to the supplement Pycnogenol, derived from French maritime pine trees. Pycnogenol has been seen to increase nitric oxide production within the arteries.

Dr Ximing Liu explained his reason for researching the potential of Pycnogenol by citing patients who no longer needed insulin to treat their type 2 diabetes. He and his associates wanted to determine whether Pycnogenol has a glucose-lowering effect. They recruited 18 men and 22 women who were outpatients at their hospital. Those subjects ranged in age from 28 to 64 and were of normal weight, overweight or obese. Patients were given 50, 100, 200, and 300mg doses of Pycnogenol in three-week intervals. Every three weeks glucose levels (both fasting and after a meal), HbA_{1C} and insulin were measured.

The researchers reported a linear, dose-dependent reduction in glucose levels up to 200mg of Pycnogenol. A 300mg dose provided no further benefit. Fasting levels were reduced from 8.64mmol/l (plus or minus 0.93) to 7.54mmol/l (plus or minus 1.64). Fifty milligrams of Pycnogenol lowered glucose levels following a meal from 12.47mmol/l (plus or minus 1.06) to 11.16mmol/l (plus or minus 2.11). Maximum decrease in glucose after a meal – at a

200mg Pycnogenol dose – was to 10.07mmol/l (plus or minus 2.69).

HbA_{1C} levels fell continuously from 8.02 per cent (plus or minus 1.04) to 7.37 per cent (plus or minus 1.09). Improvement was noted at nine to 12 weeks with 200mg or 300mg of Pycnogenol. There was no difference seen in insulin levels, indicating that beneficial changes were not due to increased insulin secretion.

The investigators did a follow-up study with 77 type-2 diabetic patients who were taking a glucose-lowering medication (hypoglycaemic agent). Once again, Pycnogenol significantly lowered blood glucose.

Though the exact mode of action by which Pycnogenol lowers blood glucose levels in diabetic patients is unknown, researchers have speculated that the powerful antioxidant supplement seems to overcome the blocked glucose uptake by cells in the body. Interestingly, in studies with diabetic rats Pycnogenol significantly lowered blood glucose while there was no such response in normal rats.

Magnesium, metabolic syndrome, diabetes and hypertension

As I explain in Chapter 9: The Electrolyte Balancing Act, it may be more important to increase and thus balance levels of minerals in the body (electrolytes) including magnesium, calcium and potassium than it is to reduce the mineral sodium in our diets. As I explain in that chapter, it's an electrolyte balancing act. It appears that magnesium may play a role in diabetes as well.

Researchers at Northwestern University, in Chicago, noted that previous studies indicated that magnesium is inversely related to risk of hypertension and type 2 diabetes; that is to say, the more magnesium in the diet, the less chance of those diseases developing. So they looked at the relationship between magnesium intake and a precursor of diabetes called the metabolic syndrome, which includes high blood pressure, overweight, inefficiency of insulin – otherwise known as 'insulin resistance' – high levels of triglycerides and lower than desired levels of the protective HDL cholesterol. Magnesium has also been observed to lower triglycerides and increase HDL.

They selected 4,637 men who were 18 to 30 years old at the start of the project and monitored them for 15 years. During that time, there were 608 cases of metabolic syndrome. Magnesium intake was inversely associated with the incidence of that syndrome. In other words, the higher the levels of magnesium in subjects, the lower the incidence of metabolic syndrome. That, in turn, can potentially reduce future incidence of diabetes.

That research was reported only in 2006. There have been no studies yet as to whether increasing magnesium consumption in the diet and by taking supplements will improve diabetes. That said, the Northwestern investigators noted that 'experimental data suggest that magnesium may directly regulate cellular glucose metabolism', and that 'magnesium intake may improve insulin sensitivity'. Both those functions of this mineral would be enormously important for diabetic people. Recommended daily intake is 500mg.

Please, please make the effort

I mentioned my friend who ignored both his doctor's advice and my urging to control his diabetes. I won't be surprised when I get the phone call that he has passed away. What a terrible waste. And in the meantime, the quality of his life is minimal.

I'll end this chapter with one more set of statistics – not to scare you but rather to encourage you to make your best possible efforts to control both your diabetes and hypertension. By all means try the lifestyle modifications including diet and exercise and give the supplements a chance. But if they don't take you all the way to solid reduction of hypertension, I urge you to work with your doctor to find the prescription medications that can save your life. Yes, those drugs can be associated with side effects. But by working with your doctor you can find one or more that will give you the reductions you need while minimising any adverse effects.

So now, the final statistics from the Centers for Disease Control and Prevention in the US, which I quote directly from the report in the *Journal of the American Medical Association*: 'If an individual is diagnosed at age 40 years, men will lose 11.6 life-years and 18.6 quality-adjusted life-years and women will lose 14.3 life-years and 22.0 quality-adjusted life-years.' Those extra years of life and quality of life are well worth working for.

Chapter 5

Take a Load Off Your Heart

Men and women are getting fatter and fatter, and we're paying the price for those super-sized meals with increased risk of blood pressure, diabetes, heart attacks and strokes. The scariest statistic I've read is that today's youngsters, who are heavier and more sedentary than ever before, will be the first generation with a life expectancy *less* than that of their parents.

When it comes to weight, we definitely are living in a global community. In the UK, 40 per cent of men and 33 per cent of women are overweight and 20 per cent are obese. Nearly two-thirds of all American men and women are overweight or obese. Statistics from the Australasian Society for the Study of Obesity indicate that more than half of all Australian women and two-thirds of men share that dubious distinction. A surgeon in the Netherlands commented that he had to put two operating tables together to operate on one heavy patient. Some patients there barely fit into scanning machines.

As people gain weight, their risk of developing hypertension grows along with them. Conversely, data show that even moderate weight loss reduces that risk. One study's investigators followed 623 middle-aged disease-free adults aged from 30 to 49 years old and 605 older adults aged 50 to 65 years. Those who lost 6.8 kg or more reduced their long-term risk of hypertension by 21 per cent while older adults losing that much weight enjoyed a 29 per cent drop in risk.

Weight gain and blood pressure are linked. The more overweight a person becomes, the higher his or her BP will be likely to go. Happily, though, the more weight an overweight individual manages to lose, the better his or her blood pressure control will be. Losing weight is, in fact, one of the most solidly documented lifestyle modifications shown to improve blood pressure.

The statistical links between weight and cardiovascular disease are totally scary. One of the most definitive studies began in 1967. Data were collected until 2002. During those years subjects were classified as normal weight, overweight or obese. The risk of being hospitalised for heart problems quadrupled in men and women after the age of 65 in the obese group. And obese individuals were more likely to die from heart attack or stroke than thinner persons.

Classifying weight and risk

We all have our own ways of discovering that we're overweight. Our clothes don't fit the way they used to. We loosen our belts a notch. Stepping on the bathroom scales isn't something we really want to do. Simple acts of movement, such as getting out of a chair, much less walking up a flight of stairs, become increasingly difficult.

But medical researchers have more precise methods of classifying overweight and obesity. The measure most often used is called the body mass index, or BMI. This gives a single figure that is based on your weight and height, regardless of your age and sex. BMI is calculated by dividing your weight in kilograms by your height in metres squared.

That is: weight (kg) ÷ height x height (m) = BMI.

For example, if you weigh 70kg (11st) and are 1.7m tall (5ft 7in) your BMI would be: $70 ÷ (1.7x1.7) = 70 ÷ 2.9 = 24$.

- Underweight is a BMI equal to or less than 19.
- Optimum or healthy weight is a BMI of 20 to 25.
- Overweight is a BMI of 25 to 30.
- Obese is a BMI equal to or greater than 30.

If maths isn't your strong point, you can use a number of BMI calculators on the internet, for example: www.core.monash.org/bmi.html.

There's one major problem with the BMI system. What about an athletic man or woman? Muscle weighs more than fat. A rugby player who stands 1.85m (6ft 1in) tall and weighs 93kg (14st 8lb) may be solid muscle with very little fat. He would scarcely be thought of as overweight, despite a BMI of 27 that would put him into that classification. A body builder might even weigh 103 kg (16st 2lb) at that same height, but he wouldn't be called obese.

Some authorities believe that changing the standard from BMI to waist-to-hip ratio would be a more accurate indicator of cardiovascular risk. That was the conclusion of the INTERHEART study involving more than 27,000 participants from 52 countries.

Others would prefer a simple measurement of waist circumference (WC) to determine weight-related health risk. This would mean:

For women:
- Optimum would be a WC of less than 80cm (32in).
- Overweight would be a WC of 80–88cm (32–35in).
- Obese would be a WC of more than 88cm (35in).

For men:
- Optimum would be a WC of less than 94cm (37in).
- Overweight would be a WC of 94–102cm (37–40in).
- Obese would be a WC of more than 102cm (40in).

I think the best approach was proposed by Canadian researchers who presented a spectrum of studies and convincingly argued for combining both BMI and WC to calculate risk. Look back at the BMI section above and work out whether your height and weight would classify you as optimum, overweight or obese. Then look at your waist circumference. Put the two together and you've got a pretty good idea of your personal risk.

Of course, I hope that you fall into the optimum weight category. But if you do, you probably wouldn't be reading this chapter other than perhaps out of curiosity.

Which diet is best?

Ultimately, the best diet is the one you'll stick with long enough not only to lose weight but also to change and improve your eating habits. It will do no good to lose that extra kilogram or so only to get it right back again along with a few more; actually, that sort of yo-yo dieting harms your body.

While there have been dozens of diet books, many of which reached the best-seller list, all fall into one category or another. Perhaps you've tried one or more of those diets.

- *Gimmick diets* advise that you concentrate on one or other food (the grapefruit or cabbage soup diets), never combine foods of different types at one time (Fit for Life and others), combine foods in a very specified manner (the Zone diet and others), alternate certain foods throughout the week, splurge after 'being good' for a few days or do some sort of fasting. The next time you might be tempted to try one of those fad diets ask yourself if you could really imagine eating that way for the rest of your life.

- *Low-carb diets* promise that you can eat all the rich foods you want, from beef to bacon to butter, but eliminate most carbohydrate-containing foods. The Atkins diet is currently the most famous of these, though they have been around for decades in one incarnation or another. As mouth-watering as this approach might sound at the start, no matter how much you love bacon and eggs pretty soon you'll be lusting for a slice of toast and marmalade and a glass of orange juice to go with that breakfast. In this diet rapid weight loss mainly comes from water loss. And studies have shown that low-carb dieters abandon the programme after no more than six months.
- *Low-fat diets* tempt dieters – and potential book buyers – with the idea that one can eat all one wants and still lose weight. Theoretically that's true, since low-fat foods typically are bulky and filling. But, as with the low-carb diets, these regimens become boring pretty fast, especially if they're vegetarian diets.

Researchers at Tufts University, in Boston, decided to put a number of diets to the test. They recruited 160 overweight or obese adults with an average BMI of 35 in an age range of 27 to 42. Subjects were put on the Atkins low-carb diet, the Zone diet of combined food specifications, the Ornish ultra-low-fat near-vegetarian diet or the Weight Watchers balanced diet that restricts calories. They were given the book that spelled out the particular diet, with no additional instruction or guidance. Participants were asked to stick with the diet for one year. But only 53 per cent stuck with Atkins, 65 per cent followed through with the Zone diet, 65 per cent with Weight Watchers, and 50 per cent with Ornish.

Weight loss was just about the same at the end of the year for all programmes, with average reductions of 2.1kg for Atkins, 3.2kg for the Zone, 3kg for Weight Watchers, and 3.3kg for Ornish. Not surprisingly, with such small weight losses, blood pressure measurements were virtually unchanged. As the authors of the study wrote, 'Overall dietary adherence rates were low, although increased adherence was associated with greater weight loss and cardiac risk factor reductions for each diet group.'

The problem with all those diets, as is true with any fad diet, is that, for virtually everyone, going on a diet means eventually coming off that diet. The only approach that really works is to change one's lifestyle enough to reduce the number of calories taken in as food and to increase the amount of calories burned through physical activity. In other words, you need to go on the 'No-Fad Diet' as Dr Robert Eckel called it in his editorial accompanying the article comparing the four diets.

The diet that works for one person won't necessarily work for you. If you absolutely love ice cream, a diet that forbids it is bound to fail. If a dinner isn't complete without a piece of bread and a glass of wine, your diet must include them both. Simply enough, you need your very own personal 'Diet for the Rest of Your Life Diet'.

Cutting through the Gordian knot

In the legend, people tried and tried to figure out a way to unravel an intricately woven knot. He who did so would be named king. Finally, Alexander the Great simply walked up and sliced through the knot with a single stroke of his sword.

Ultimately, weight control can be likened to that Gordian knot. We can slice through all the complications and gimmicks to reveal the essential knowledge needed to lose weight, maintain that weight loss and remain healthy, while lowering BP, very simply. There are certain foods we want to eat a lot of and others we should limit. No radical gimmickry here, just straightforward logic, like cutting through that knot.

Foods to emphasise in the diet provide a lot of nutrients as well as fibre and protective plant substances called polyphenols. These include fruits, vegetables and wholegrain bread and cereals. To those, add at least two portions (and preferably three or even four) of fish and other seafood, especially oily fish rich in omega-3 fatty acids, which are so good for our hearts. But there's no reason to eliminate red meat. Just choose the leanest cuts of beef, pork, lamb and veal. Try to have two or three daily servings of fat-free or low-fat dairy foods – not just milk but also yogurt and cheese – for their calcium and other nutrients. Enjoy nuts in moderation as a healthy snack. And choose lots of dishes made from beans and peas that provide soluble fibre to lower cholesterol and improve BP. For weight management purposes, go easy on all types of oil. While they may be healthy, they work out at 110 calories per tablespoon.

Foods to limit or even avoid – at least while trying to lose weight – are those that provide little or no nutritional value but represent a lot of empty calories. In restaurants, ask the waiter or waitress not to bring a bread basket. Avoid that temptation entirely. And limit white bread at home. Each slice you give up knocks at least 100 calories from your daily intake. The same goes for pasta and rice. Sure they're delicious, but offer nothing but calories. Needless to say, those trying to lose weight should virtually eliminate cakes, sweets, biscuits and other high-calorie confections. At the very least, opt for the smallest portions of such high-cal treats. After dinner in the evening, a steaming mug of hot cocoa made with calorie-free sweetener such as sucralose (Splenda) is relaxing, comforting, and satisfying – without the calories.

Really and truly, that's all the nutrition advice, in a nutshell, you need to very successfully lose weight and ultimately maintain healthy weight and blood pressure for the rest of your life. And it'll be a longer, more enjoyable life.

Start writing your own diet book

I mean that quite literally. The best way to begin a successful weight loss, and ultimately life-long weight control, programme is to critically analyse what you're eating and drinking, to learn what foods and beverages are keeping you overweight. I suggest that you start writing a daily diary or journal.

Record everything – and I do mean everything – you eat and drink and when you consume those foods and beverages. The closer you get to being your personal researcher the better. Don't just jot down that you 'had a soft drink in the afternoon'. Specify what kind of drink and how much you drank. Invest in kitchen scales you can use to weigh those servings of food. Was it a 250ml glass or a half-litre bottle? Was it a 100g steak or a half kilo? Did you snack on 'a few' nuts or the entire packet? Start paying attention to the calories in the foods you eat. Be totally honest with yourself.

Keep that food and drink diary for a full week, eating as you normally do and not trying to take a short cut or fool yourself. I hope you're not the sort of person who cheats at solitaire!

After a week of scrupulous note taking, read and critique your eating and drinking habits. Look at that diary as though it were written by someone else. Put yourself into the role of dietitian. Where would it be fairly painless to cut back on serving sizes? A glass of red wine with a small lean steak for dinner protects against cardiovascular disease in a delicious way. But a full bottle washing down a half-kilo chunk of well-marbled beef may be a bit excessive, don't you agree? What foods provide lots of calories with little or no nutrient value? When are you snacking? While watching TV in the evening after a stressful day?

What are the changes you're willing to make and what eating habits would you fight to the death for? Simply must have that bowl of ice cream in the evening? Not a problem. But could you switch to a low-fat brand, reduce the serving size by probably half, and top the dessert off with some fresh berries? Could you make that slice of toast in the morning wholegrain, and spread it with a scrape of soft margarine and a dab of low-cal preserve? If watching TV in the living room or the family room downstairs prompts you to gorge on snacks, could you go upstairs and read a book instead, thus breaking the Pavlovian connection? Or could you plan in advance to have snacks that won't expand your waistline? Perhaps a platter of freshly sliced oranges and apples? Or some fat-free, sugar-free popcorn or pretzels?

Only you can make the choices you'll be able to live with. And don't try to change everything at once. Little things can truly mean a lot. I'm always reminded when I write or speak about such things of the day my late father-in-law, Ben, told the family he was going to shed the one-stone spare tyre around his waist by not putting sugar in his coffee.

Everyone laughed, thinking such an insignificant thing couldn't possibly make a difference, especially a one-stone difference.

But think about the numbers. One teaspoon of sugar has 16 calories. Ben added three spoons to his coffee and drank five cups daily. Multiply three teaspoons by 16 and then multiply those 48 calories by five cups for a total of 240 calories a day, 7,200 calories a month. That number of calories yields two pounds of weight loss or gain. In seven months, Ben lost that stone in weight without doing anything else!

Pre-emptive snacking

No matter what sort of diet you follow in order to lose weight, and I'll discuss those options in the coming pages, I have a tip that's certain to help. It all began with research carried out in the 1960s at Michigan State University. The study was very simple, especially when compared with the complex projects of today. Women who wanted to lose weight were given just one instruction: 20 to 30 minutes before meals, they were to eat a slice of wholegrain bread. Participants in the study who followed that advice lost weight in a very satisfying manner.

How and why did that simple change work? As we eat, food is converted to blood sugar, glucose, that enters the blood stream to provide energy for the body. It takes about 20 minutes for sensors in the brain to pick up the fact that blood sugar levels have risen and that there isn't any need for more food. As those glucose levels rise, we're no longer hungry. The problem is that when we're really hungry and start to eat, we don't give the body and brain time to recognise the fact that sugar levels have gone up. We shouldn't be hungry any longer, but we continue to eat.

By eating that slice of bread 20 to 30 minutes before lunch and dinner, women in the MSU study caused their blood sugar levels to rise before they sat down to eat their meal. When they did so, they weren't as hungry and didn't eat as much as they would have done otherwise. They lost weight.

I put this into practice when my children were little. I was trying to establish a heart-healthy lifestyle to protect them from heart disease later in life. That meant limiting the cake, biscuits, ice cream, pizza and so on that they consumed. So when they were invited to birthday parties or elsewhere, about 20 minutes before we were to leave the house I'd ask if they were hungry. Of course little kids are always hungry! So I'd give them a healthy snack of some sliced fruit, a small sandwich, a cup of soup or something like that. When they got to the party, they weren't ravenous and therefore ate a lot less fatty food than they would have done otherwise.

Many individuals have practised this 'pre-emptive snacking' without realising it. Whoever is preparing the evening's meal will frequently taste foods while cooking. While peeling the carrots, most of us will eat one or two pieces. When setting out the bread, both my wife and I tend to break off the knob and eat it. Do that a few times and blood sugar begins to rise and one isn't as hungry when dinner is served to the rest of the family.

Make pre-emptive snacking part of your lifestyle. Start with breakfast. If you're not in a hurry to get out of the house, drink your glass of juice or have a slice of toast with the first cup of coffee 20 to 30 minutes before sitting down to the full meal. If you've taken a lunch box to work, you won't overeat since there'll only be a limited amount of food in that box. But if you're heading out for lunch, remember to have that snack before you leave.

Ultimately, the ideal would be to never get very hungry. Make sure you have another healthy snack mid-afternoon. That doesn't mean a typical doughnut or muffin and coffee. Instead make it a handful of nuts or dried fruit or perhaps a cereal bar.

The evening meal offers the most temptation to overeat. Rather than waiting for dinner to be served, whether you're cooking it or not, get into the healthy habit of eating a rather substantial snack well before dinner. I personally enjoy some herring on wholegrain crackers. Or I might have a pot of yogurt. I keep bite-size pre-cut vegetables, or *crudités*, in the refrigerator to munch on while watching the evening news while my wife prepares dinner (or while I prepare dinner, if it's my turn to cook).

Give pre-emptive snacking a try for a couple of weeks and see if that doesn't make you eat less at major meals. To be most successful, keep a supply of healthy snacks on hand so that they're readily available.

Avoid stress eating

I love living in this modern age with all its wonderful advances and advantages. But stress is part and parcel of life for most of us. The higher the level of stress during the day, the more likely we'll use food in the evening as a coping mechanism. We eat continuously not because we're hungry but simply as a nervous instinct. I suppose it's a better habit than self-medicating into anaesthesia with booze, but it's still not very healthy.

The emphasis in that last sentence should be on the word 'habit'. We get into a deeply embedded habit of non-stop eating in the evening, especially when watching television or a DVD. Fortunately there are a few ways to deal with that bad habit.

The easiest approach is to accept the habit and simply try to modify it a bit. Think about your own evening snacking. If you're like most people, you head for the refrigerator or the larder and grab the first food you see. If that food happens to be salty potato crisps (or 'chips' as we Americans call them), that's what you'll eat. And very likely you'll devour the entire bag. Instead of serving yourself a small bowl of ice cream, you'll take the tub out and dig in with a spoon, sometimes until there's no more ice cream left.

Let's modify those habits. What if those crisps weren't in the larder at all, and instead you find some nuts in their shells? Put a handful or two in a bowl along with a nut-cracker and crack open the nuts as you sit in front of the TV. The idea is to keep your hands busy shelling the nuts rather than eating ready shelled nuts out of a packet.

Make your own popcorn from scratch rather than use the microwaveable types that are loaded with trans-fatty acids. The aromas that fill the house are wonderful and put you into a much more relaxed mood.

An alternative that I strongly prefer is making a steaming cup of hot cocoa. Low in fat and calories, that cup of cocoa relaxes the mind and can help lower blood pressure thanks to its polyphenol content. See the recipes in Chapter 17 for preparation tips. I personally find I get a much better night's sleep after a mug of cocoa.

As a complete alternative to snacking, keep one of those squeezable rubber balls or worry beads or something else to keep your hands busy instead of eating. Try putting a couple of lightweight dumb-bells next to the couch or chair and keep busy doing some exercise.

Or try to break the conditioned response entirely. In a way, many of us are like Pavlov's dogs, conditioned to snack when we sit in our established chair or couch and the TV goes on. To break the habit, read a book or a magazine. Don't turn the TV on at all.

Perhaps play some music. You'll need both hands to hold that book or magazine. And since you're not in the habit of snacking while reading, you probably won't.

I have a personal house rule that calls for zero food or drink in the bedroom. Knowing that I'll snack, sometimes to excess, when I'm under stress and watching TV, I'll head upstairs to the bedroom instead. There I'll either do some reading or TV viewing. But I'm 'conditioned' not to eat in that room. Think about your own snacking and 'conditioning', and deliberately work to reverse those behavioural patterns.

The *dim sum* diet

Dim sum is a wonderful and interesting way to enjoy Chinese food. Essentially, *dim sum* is a variety of different foods served in small quantities on little plates. The waiter comes along with a trolley offering this food or that. You either choose to have it or pass. As you eat the foods, which come on different coloured dishes that reflect the price, plates pile up on the table and at the end of the meal the price is determined by adding up the number of those plates.

What I suggest for what I call the '*dim sum* diet' has nothing to do with Chinese food other than the concept of having small servings of this and that. And there's even some solid science behind the idea.

The weight loss clinic at University of California at Los Angeles (UCLA) medical school uses a similar approach. They have developed meal substitutes that come in individual servings and a variety of flavours to be mixed with water or diet soda. Each of those packets provide exactly 100 calories and a balance of protein, fat, and carbohydrate. Dieters are instructed to eat eight to nine meal substitutes throughout the day. The very low calorie intake, of course, facilitates rapid and satisfying weight loss. And by having a mini-meal every two hours, dieters report – much to their amazement – that they are never hungry.

In my version, I combine the best of the UCLA thinking with the unusual Chinese approach to dining out. Instead of meal substitutes, my *dim sum* diet calls for a wide variety of foods eaten throughout the day that have about 100 calories each. Eat eight to nine times a day. You can combine two 100-calorie selections if you wish, but do so no more than twice daily. In addition to those foods, you can also have all the salad greens you can eat dressed with a squeeze of lemon or lime, a splash of flavoured vinegar such as balsamic or a tablespoon of low-cal dressing. Since your food intake will be quite limited, supplement with a multivitamin/mineral tablet. Here's a list of some foods that you might consider.

Dim sum diet foods	Serving size	Calories
Seafood		
Salmon	56g	125
Halibut	112g	84
Cooked prawns	74g	100
Scallops	112g	92
Tuna	56g	96

Dim sum diet foods	Serving size	Calories
Poultry		
Chicken breast	112g	100
Turkey burger	70g	100
Egg salad	112g	100
Beef		
Extra lean beef burger	56g	100
Roast beef	70g	111
95% fat-free hot dog	1	54
Pork		
Bacon	2 slices	89
Grilled pork chop	100g	150
Lean ham	100g	100
Egg (boiled)	1 large	78
Dairy		
Skimmed milk	240ml	86
Plain yogurt	200ml	170
Cottage cheese	30g	30
Cheddar cheese (low-fat)	30ml	55
Vegetables		
Tomato	88g	27
Carrots	1 medium	31
Broccoli (raw)	120ml	12
Cauliflower (raw)	120ml	13
Peppers (chopped)	50g	14
Fruit		
Apple	1 medium	138

Dim sum diet foods	Serving size	Calories
Banana	1 medium	114
Grapefruit	½ medium	118
Kiwi fruit	1 medium	76
Peach	1 medium	37
Mango	½ medium	103
Pear	1 medium	98
Nuts		
Dry roasted almonds	15g	83
Cashews	15g	82
Peanuts	15g	83
Walnuts	15g	86

Spend a little time at the supermarket and read the labels of other potential foods for the *dim sum* diet. Check out the calories and serving sizes of soups, tinned stews and chilli con carne, sardines, tinned fish, such as salmon and tuna, that you can eat from the tin, bread and cereals, and other items that you'd enjoy. The wider the variety of foods you eat during the weight loss period the better so that you don't get bored.

This diet is especially convenient for those who live on their own or with those who have a different eating pattern. An extra benefit is the time saved by not having to prepare meals.

As with any diet, it's best to avoid alcoholic drinks – for two reasons. First, they're obviously a source of calories. Second, they relax inhibitions and might lead you to eat more than you really want to. That said, when my wife went on the diet to lose a few pounds before we headed off on holiday she replaced one of the mini-meals with a glass of wine in the evening. A 150ml serving has about 100 calories. If you'd prefer a cocktail in the evening, a 55ml tumbler of the spirit of your choice – gin, vodka, rum – has 90 calories. Mix with diet cola, soda water or plain water.

This is a rather unusual approach to dieting, I think you'll agree. UCLA has had tremendous success, whether subjects wanted to lose 4 or 40 kg. To lose very large amounts of weight, obese individuals have followed the programme for up to a full year.

Does my *dim sum* diet fall into the category of 'gimmick' diets as I categorised diets above? You bet. On the other hand there's a lot of UCLA research behind its development. It's a different approach that some people will find helpful.

The breakfast cereal diet

Here's another 'gimmick' diet, but, again, it's been shown to work. The breakfast cereal diet calls for eating one serving (typically 150–200g) of any ready-to-eat cold cereal with 160ml of skimmed milk and 300g of berries – which would add about 100 calories for breakfast – and again for either lunch or dinner. Since dinner typically packs in far more calories than lunch, that would probably be more effective. One would eat a normal meal once daily, for either lunch or dinner.

A study showed that overweight and obese men and women who followed this plan for two weeks lost 1–2kg. The control group, eating normally, lost just 30g or so.

Until recently I never knew this was a formally designated diet. I've been replacing an evening meal once in a while with breakfast cereal for years. It saves time and, for me, is an easy way to lose just a pound or two when I might need to do so.

Learning portion control

Virtually every country in the world has developed a guide to healthy eating. Most call for eating a wide variety of foods daily to ensure getting all the nutrients needed.

The foundation of a healthy diet should be a minimum of

five portions of fruits and vegetables daily. Personally I think, and many, if not most, authorities agree, that the minimum should be up to nine servings a day. You might think that's a huge amount, but two things come into play. First plant-based foods pack in very few calories per serving. And a serving is a lot less than the average person might guess.

A portion of fruit, as defined by nutritionists, might be one medium apple, banana, pear or peach. Or it could be two figs or 15 grapes or 100g of berries or 100ml of apple sauce. A portion of dried fruit would be two tablespoons of raisins or two medium plums (prunes) or four apple rings. Just 175ml of fruit juice constitutes a serving. Starting the day with a glass of juice and some cold cereal with a sliced banana and 100g of berries gives you three servings right off the bat. Grab some raisins or prunes for a snack and you're up to four. Then maybe sliced mango for dessert at dinner to total five fruit portions for the day.

And what about vegetables? Similarly small amounts constitute a portion. For raw veggies it's 100g. A serving of tomato juice or other vegetable juice is 120ml. A serving of any cooked vegetables would be just 112 grams. A bowl of soup typically will contain two vegetable portions. What you would probably think to be one serving when you'd see vegetables on a plate would likely be two or, in restaurants, perhaps even three.

The one thing that has shown up in medical studies time and time again, with no contradictory evidence, is that those whose diets are rich in fruits and vegetables get some protection against cardiovascular disease, have lower blood pressure, and suffer fewer heart attacks and strokes.

The same holds for wholegrain bread and cereals. Most food guides call for three to four portions daily. In terms of weight control, limit the amount of foods in this category made with refined flour, including pasta, white bread, cakes and dessert items. Bear in mind that a serving of cooked pasta is 140g, which has about 200 calories, not the huge 400g mounds one often sees.

Start thinking the same way about meat and dairy foods. A portion of meat of any kind is 100g, about the size of a pack of playing cards or a man's palm. A half-kilo steak is *not* one portion! A serving of cheese of any variety is 28g. Picture a 2.5cm (1in) square chunk of cheddar, fontina or Swiss cheese.

Simply learning to judge serving sizes and eating accordingly will help you to lose weight and to maintain that weight loss. Remember that it's a matter of life-long change of eating habits, not just weight loss that rebounds within a few months.

The essential weight control ingredient

This will be the shortest section in this chapter. Simply stated, weight loss and subsequent weight maintenance *requires* physical activity. It's not an option. It is absolutely essential. Every study I've ever read that investigates long-term weight control concludes that regular, fairly strenuous physical activity must go hand in hand with limiting calories.

In our modern society, we have become rather like livestock being fattened for the market, with limited movement and unlimited feed. The process by which a previously fit individual becomes overweight and possibly obese is gradual and quite insidious. As one becomes sedentary, muscle slowly gets replaced by fat. At first, a person thinks all's well when he or she looks down at the bathroom scales. But, like a well-marbled slab of beef, that person becomes fatter and less muscular.

The only tissue in our bodies capable of burning significant numbers of calories is muscle. Neither skin nor bone nor fat burns much energy in comparison. Muscle tissue is the furnace of our bodies. As the percentage of muscle decreases, the ability to expend energy decreases as well. One day, the sedentary individual who has not changed dietary habits by a single calorie since the time he or she was physically fit begins to gain weight. 'But doctor,' such patients complain, 'I'm not eating any more food than I ever have.' And that's true. But there isn't enough muscle left to burn those same calories. And weight goes up and up and up.

Enough said. It's time to add a regimen of physical activity to your lifestyle. It's so important that I've written an entire chapter in this book.

Go ahead, step on your bathroom scales

Diet experts have argued about this one for years, as long as I've been writing about health and medical matters. Whoops, make that decades instead of years! Some have advised those trying to lose weight to weigh themselves only once a week. Others recommended a weigh-in every three or four days. Their reasoning was twofold. First, weight loss is a rather slow process and men and women could get discouraged. Second, weight varies slightly from hour to hour and day to day. Thus seeing a ½-kilo gain could scuttle a diet.

But two separate recent studies have determined that daily weighing is the 'weigh to go' both for weight loss and maintenance. In the first study, carried out at the University of Minnesota, researchers monitored 3,000 overweight or obese men and women for two to three years. Half were in a weight loss programme while the other half were in a programme to prevent weight gain. Individuals in the weight-loss programme, who weighed themselves daily, lost twice as much weight as those who weighed themselves only weekly. The difference was impressive: 5.45kg compared with 2.7kg respectively. And those who never weighed themselves *gained* about 1.8kg on average over the course of two years. Conversely, subjects in the weight gain prevention programme who weighed themselves daily *lost* weight.

Researchers in the second study at the Weight Control

Center, at Brown University, Rhode Island, tracked 291 men and women on a weight-maintenance programme for 17 months, following an average weight loss of 10 per cent of body weight. Of those who did daily weigh-ins, 39 per cent lost at least 2.3kg. That was as good as or better than subjects participating in support groups. And it was vastly superior to those who weighed themselves less often than daily; 68 per cent regained at least 2.3kg.

It's really very simple and logical when one thinks about it. Step on the scales at about the same time of day every day. If you see a slight weight gain, even though that might be due to a normal daily fluctuation, you'll cut back on the day's food intake. By the next day you'll likely see that unwanted weight gone. That, in turn, encourages a person to remain diligent in their weight control efforts.

Make the small investment needed to purchase good-quality scales. Weigh yourself each and every day as part of your weight control and blood pressure control programme.

Icing on the cake

Well, that might not be the proper metaphor in discussing this particular subject but there are many benefits to weight loss beyond good health and blood pressure control, as vitally important as those are. You'll relish hearing friends, relatives, and work colleagues tell you how much better you look. Buying new clothes becomes something to look forward to. You'll sleep better, have more energy, experience fewer mid-afternoon slumps, and simply enjoy life a lot more.

Chapter 6

Pressure-Friendly Active Lifestyle

There's a single element found in successful weight loss, cholesterol control, stress management, diabetes prevention, and blood pressure maintenance. It's something virtually everyone all over the world who has enjoyed a long life has in common. In fact, it is the one factor that all medical authorities agree is essential for both quality and quantity of life. What is this 'snake oil' that appears to be the 'cure for what ails you'? It's physical activity.

Note that I didn't use the term 'exercise'. The healthiest men and women in the world aren't necessarily the ones heading off to the gym, but rather those who are physically active most days if not all days of the week. That's not to say that you should quit your membership of the gym or health club if you enjoy working out on the treadmill or rowing machine or doing aerobics. My wife, for example, lives a relatively sedentary life as a high school English teacher and in her leisure time plays duplicate bridge. She really doesn't enjoy the outdoors the way I do, but she likes taking exercise classes at the health club. One day she'll do a cycle class, another day it'll be an aerobics class combined with strength and flexibility training. The only sport she loves is skiing, which we do together whenever we can.

On the other hand, I can't wait to get outdoors whenever I can. I love to hike, to ride a bicycle, to ski in our local mountains, and, most frequently, to walk the up-and-down hills of the golf courses in the canyons where we live. When travelling on business or for pleasure, there's nothing I enjoy more than exploring a new place by walking, often for three or four or more miles. That said, my work schedule doesn't permit me to do those kinds of recreational activities except at weekends and on holiday. Most days of the week I 'condense' my activity in the gym, where I walk the treadmill or ride the exercise bike while watching the morning news on a TV screen.

There are many ways of staying fit and of getting the physical activity we all need for good health in general and good heart health in particular. Even if you're absolutely set against exercise, whether called physical activity or something else, and define yourself as the ultimate couch potato, please bear with me through this short chapter. To begin with, I can really relate to you. As a kid in elementary school in the fifties I flunked the president's physical fitness test while almost everyone else passed. I was always the last one picked for any team sport. No, I am not now nor have I ever been an athlete who is naturally attracted to fitness and exercise.

To make matters worse, I went to college in the 1960s, a truly self-destructive era. No one exercised. If anyone was running on campus, you could assume that a cop was chasing him! And after college I became a typical American sedentary office worker.

Looking back on those days, I realise that I was always tired and never felt really well. Yawning every afternoon. Nodding off in meetings, even interesting ones. Not sleeping well at night and having a tough time getting up in the mornings. Lousy at sports – I got into skiing not for the sport but rather for the opportunity to meet girls in the lodge at night. In those days I was actually happy when bad weather kept us off the slopes and in the lodge. I did a lot better with the girls playing my guitar inside than skiing, since I was just too weak to do fancy turns and skied out of control and fell over a lot.

When I had my heart attack and first bypass surgery in 1978 at the tender age of 35, there was no such thing as cardiac rehabilitation and I got no advice about exercise. So if I did anything strenuous I was scared that I'd have another heart attack.

Then, in 1984, my life changed. On 3 July I had my second bypass operation, and three weeks later my cardiologist had me – much against my will – in a rehab programme. Little by little I came to life: walking slowly on the treadmill, riding slowly on the bicycle. Everything I did at the beginning I did slowly. But by the end of just six weeks, I was feeling better than at any time I could recall. By the end of the 12-week programme, I was well on my way to enjoying a life of fitness that I'd never experienced before.

I came to revel in being able to do things that I thought only 'sporty types' could do. And on my first ski trip, a year later, I found that, much to my surprise, I could actually ski. I was physically able to do the things that I'd learned in lessons before. It was fun! It was as though I had a brand-new body.

So, there you are. You're not reading the advice of some Olympic athlete or a wild-eyed fanatic. Put simply, if I can make the transformation, anyone can!

Looking at things in retrospect, it's too bad it took such a near-catastrophic illness to turn me around. I think of all those years I could have enjoyed more. Sooner would have been better than later, but later was better than never. And now I swear I'll never go back to the old ways. Life is a lot more fun when you have the energy to enjoy it.

Activate your healthy heart
This isn't a book for sick people. It's for those who want to prevent problems and for those who want to enjoy their health

and their life. But the one thing that I learned in cardiac rehab that applies to a programme of physical fitness for everyone is the word 'slowly'. It took years to get to your current level of sedentary behaviour and lack of fitness, and it'll take time to get going. How long? Ninety days. Give yourself just 90 days. Make a promise, a commitment, to follow the advice in this chapter and I promise, in turn, that by the end of that time you'll be converted for life. You won't want to give up the way you'll feel.

Whether you're trying to prevent a heart attack or stroke or you want to avoid a second one, exercise just has to be an integral part of the programme. Yet the word 'exercise' is itself enough to turn off most people. I can say that because the fact is that the vast majority of men and women in the US, the UK, Canada, Australia and New Zealand, and the rest of the Western world, are almost totally sedentary. Thanks to the remote control, they don't even have to walk to the TV to change channels. If you're one of those, you'll be please to know that you don't need to exercise in the 'no pain no gain' or 'go for the burn' sense of the term. You just need to get active, to just move your body.

Researchers at the Aerobics Institute, in Dallas, Texas, wanted to know just how fit people had to be to prevent degenerative diseases including heart disease. Dr Steven Blair and his associates studied thousands of men and women, putting them into one of five categories of fitness and regular activity. He expected to see a linear increase in health, a bigger pay-off, with every increment of exercise. The results were amazing.

To no one's surprise, those in the top category of fitness were the healthiest. But those in the second-from-bottom level, just above the truly sedentary couch potatoes who did absolutely nothing, got almost as much benefit from a minimum amount of activity as those in the top tier. The lesson learned: it doesn't take much effort to protect your health adequately.

But how can one measure the activity needed to achieve health and vitality and to prevent heart disease and stroke and other diseases, including hypertension?

In the past, people were forever talking about heart rates and measuring their pulses. That's really not very practical. Who wants to become obsessed with measuring their heartbeat while walking down the street or riding a bicycle at the weekend or, even more to the point, when dancing to a fast beat? And, it turns out, that's not at all necessary. The trick to effective physical activity comes down to a concept known for many years by exercise physiologists, but seldom shared with the rest of the world. It's a way of thinking about activity known as METs, and it's really simple.

When you're completely relaxed, just sitting in a chair quietly or lying in bed or on a couch watching television, you're burning just enough energy to keep your internal organs operating and your body alive. That amount of energy, regardless of your age, sex, height or weight, is one metabolic unit of activity, one MET. It's the lowest metabolic level of activity. Get up from that chair to open the window or find a snack, and you've stoked up your body's furnace to two METs.

The thinking behind the MET is very logical and easy to understand. When we engage in any physical activity, the heart beats to match demand, to pump out the amount of oxygen-carrying blood needed. Some activities require 50 per cent of an individual's maximal capacity. Others call for 60 per cent. Still others may need even more. You can determine your own maximum capacity very easily. Simply subtract your age from the number 220. The result is the maximum heart rate per minute you can achieve without harm. Obviously, we must never reach that maximum output.

Let's say you're 40 years old. Subtracting 40 from 220 leaves 180. That's your maximum. Normal heart rate, on average, is about 70. So you'd have a long way to go to reach your maximum capacity. Walking briskly might bring your heart rate up to 100 beats per minute. That would be 55 per cent of your maximum capacity.

At the same time, our lungs pump oxygen-rich air in and carbon dioxide-laden air out. Again, we have maximum capacities for vigorous breathing. The scientific term for this is VO2max, referring to the maximum volume of oxygen we can accommodate. That's all you need to know.

Put the two – heart rate and breathing rate – together and you have a measure of physical performance or level of activity. This measure is termed the 'metabolic equivalent', or MET. Virtually every human activity can be categorised according to the effort required, measured in METs. Take a look at the table on page 91 for a list of daily activities and their MET ratings.

Remember that I said that *activity* not *exercise* is the key to health and fitness. Virtually all medical authorities today agree that walking briskly for 30 to 40 minutes a day, at between three and four miles per hour, is sufficient daily exercise. That means about two miles a day, 14 miles a week. Do just that little bit, or its equivalent, daily and your heart will thank you for it. That walk will burn from four to six METs. You can get the same benefit by performing activities requiring half the METs for twice the time or those requiring twice the METs for half the time.

Maybe it's a very busy day, and you just don't have time to take that 30-to-40-minute walk. Studies have shown that we can break it down to ten- to 15-minute chunks of time. The benefit accumulates throughout the day. Or you might concentrate on activities that require the same METs: climbing the stairs instead of using the lift; picking up the pace when doing housework; stepping lively when you need to get from one place to another, whether from your car to an office through the car park, down the corridor from one office to another, shopping for groceries, or fetching the dry cleaning.

Vacuuming the carpet or mopping the floor can be pretty boring. Here's a tip to make those chores less onerous and good for your heart at the same time. Put on some fast-paced music. Maybe swing music, polka or hip-hop – whatever you like that gets your toe tapping. Now, instead of dancing to that music, do your chores to the beat. Suddenly you're exercising! You're activating your healthy heart!

Yes, I said that measuring your heart rate isn't necessary. But just to prove a point, place a finger on the side of your neck, just under your jaw, while you're doing some of those relatively low-MET activities. You'll find that your heart is beating faster – and you're breathing more deeply – than when you're at rest.

Conversely, you can get the benefit of a low-MET activity by doing activities requiring twice the METs for half the time. Instead of walking at four miles per hour for 40 minutes, you can jog at five to six miles per hour for 20 minutes. It's your choice. Hate to jog but love to dance? Get into the habit of square dancing or folk dancing or swing dancing on a regular basis.

Did you play with a skipping rope when you were a kid? That's one of the best forms of cardio exercise. Sound sort of sissy? Think of those boxers training in the gym; every single boxer skips. Do you want to call them sissies to their face? I think not. Forget those infomercials with expensive, inconvenient equipment. You can easily carry a skipping rope wherever you go. Take one with you during travel for business or pleasure. Keep one in the office for when you have just five minutes to get in some physical activity. For best results, buy a good-quality rope suited to your height at a sporting goods store.

Most people think that medicine has to taste bad to be effective. They apply that same thinking to activities, concentrating on what might be distasteful to them, what they would call 'exercise'. Instead, concentrate on the things that are fun for you, whether that might be riding a horse, pedalling a bicycle, rowing a boat, paddling a canoe or gardening.

Why bother to make the effort?

I could cite chapter and verse from the scientific literature to try to make a convincing argument for the health benefits of exercise. Just lifting the many volumes of books and journals would be a lot of exercise in itself. I'll spare you the details, but here are some of the benefits of regular physical activity.

You'll feel better

Whatever activity you choose, when the heart and breathing rate increase to the point that you're breathing deeply and have at least a little perspiration, your body produces a soothing substance called beta-endorphin chemically related to morphine. Its calming effect can last the entire day.

You'll feel less stressed

Most psychologists recognise physical activity as one of the best ways to reduce stress. Especially when done on a regular basis, exercise can and will enable you to cope with stress more effectively.

You'll sleep better

Exercise promotes the release of another chemical, a neurotransmitter known as serotonin. In fact, pharmaceutical companies keep trying to develop drugs that increase serotonin levels to sell as tranquillisers. Exercise is a natural way to produce serotonin to ensure better sleep at night.

You'll be more productive at work

Most people feel sleepy by mid-afternoon. Those who regularly exercise find that mid-day slumps are a thing of the past. Their stamina increases along with their ability to concentrate. In a survey of highly successful men and women in a number of professions, Dr Kenneth Pelletier, of Stanford University, found that virtually all had a regular schedule of physical activity and that they credited their productivity to their exercise habits.

You'll enjoy sports and leisure recreation more

Whether you play golf or tennis or any other sport, you'll find that you do it better and enjoy it more when you get regular exercise rather than being a 'weekend warrior'. That'll probably result in your playing those sports more often and getting even more exercise and getting even better.

You'll live longer

Here's a little detail that most people find at least moderately interesting. Study after study has shown that physical fitness prolongs life. The more strenuous the activity the longer one is likely to live.

You'll control your weight more easily and be able to eat more

Not only do you burn calories during physical activity, but also the body's metabolism remains revved up for hours afterwards. In addition, as fitness levels increase, you'll build more lean muscle. Since only muscle can burn significant numbers of calories, acting as the body's furnace, you'll be able to consume more food without gaining weight. You'll find out more about this in Chapter 5.

You'll stabilise blood sugar levels and help control diabetes

Along with weight loss, regular physical activity can virtually eliminate the symptoms and health hazards of type 2, non-insulin-dependent diabetes. Exercise has an insulin-like effect.

You'll be less likely to form blood clots that can trigger heart attack and stroke

In sedentary individuals, sudden bursts of activity can cause blood clotting. That may explain why people have heart attacks when doing unaccustomed activities such as sweeping leaves, shovelling snow or playing a strenuous sport at the weekend. But active men and women are protected against this tendency of blood platelets to form clots. Again, the more one exercises, the greater the protection.

You'll turn back your body clock

Studies have shown that regular physical activity prevents age-related decline in strength and stamina. For sedentary individuals, six months of endurance exercise reversed 30 years of decline.

Actively lower your blood pressure

Not only can regular physical activity help to lower blood pressure, but it also takes very little to achieve significant improvements. To determine just how much benefit one can expect, doctors at Tulane University, in New Orleans, examined the data from 54 studies involving a total of 2,419 men and women. Aerobic exercise was associated with what researchers called 'impressive' reductions of nearly 4 points in systolic BP and 3 points diastolic BP on average. The higher one's blood pressure at the start of an exercise programme, the greater the improvements. But everyone benefits, whether BP is high or normal, and regardless of weight or ethnic origin.

In an editorial published in *The Lancet*, New Zealand doctors summarised what we know about activity levels and blood pressure. Here are the highlights of their summary.

- There were improvements in resting heart rate, total cholesterol, LDL cholesterol, and both systolic and diastolic blood pressure after just six weeks, as reported in a 2005 report.
- One session of exercise at just 40 per cent of maximum capacity, the equivalent of moderate walking, can lower blood pressure significantly for up to 24 hours.
- After three consecutive periods of activity, let's say three days of moderate walking, blood pressure is reduced for days, returning to pre-exercise levels only after a week or two of no exercise.
- Blood pressure falls further in hypertensive individuals than those with normal BP or pre-hypertension. Those with hypertension can lower their systolic BP by 11 points and diastolic BP by 8 points, on average.
- Exercise can slash ten-year risk of heart attack and stroke by at least 25 per cent in the average hypertensive patient, because of the effect on blood pressure and other cardiovascular risk factors.
- Exercising just three times a week, for between 30 and 60 minutes a day, is as effective for lowering BP as exercising five times weekly.
- Breaking down one's physical activities into ten-minute segments is also effective. You don't need to exercise continuously for 30 minutes or more at a time.
- Aerobic exercise (walking, cycling and so on) appears to be more effective at lowering BP than resistance exercise (such as weight lifting).
- 'Low-to-moderate intensities of exercise are as effective at lowering blood pressure, if not more effective, than vigorous exercise,' was the article's conclusion.

So how does physical activity result in such outstanding pay-offs? It improves blood flow to the heart, arterial flexibility and arterial function. It slows the development of atherosclerosis and reduces the risk of heart attack and stroke.

Taking baby steps

The ancient Chinese proverb that a journey of one thousand miles begins with a single step has special meaning for those who want to get their BP down. In fact, the worst thing one could do would be to put on a pair of trainers and go out for a five-mile jog. Start slowly but surely.

If you have been sedentary for many years, and especially if you're overweight, be sure to talk to your doctor before starting any exercise programme. Regardless of your current physical condition, he or she will be delighted to have you increase your activity level and will provide personal guidelines for you.

Consider buying an inexpensive pedometer, one of those little devices worn on a belt, to determine the distance covered in numbers of steps, miles or kilometres. Start wearing it right away. I think you'll be surprised at how many steps you take during a normal day's activities, without any effort to do more. Using that number as a benchmark, gradually increase your activity.

Your goal would be to increase the number of steps taken each day to 10,000. Remember that all steps count, whether you're out for a brisk walk or simply climbing a flight of stairs at home or work. Wearing that pedometer acts as a reminder and a motivator. Most men and women find it fun to see each day's improvement over the last.

The steps you take start to add up pretty quickly, especially when you make a conscious effort. You'll take more steps when you park your car at the most distant spot when you go shopping. Park your car a street away from work, instead of right at the workplace. Then make it two streets. Then three and so on. Take the stairs instead of the lift as often as possible. Instead of sitting over a cup of tea or coffee at your break, go out for a brisk ten-minute walk.

Make those steps as much fun as possible. Here's one suggestion for golfers who normally ride a golf cart. After your drive from the tee, let your buddy take the golf cart while you walk to the ball with a couple of clubs to take your next shot. On par threes, hit the ball and then walk with (hopefully) your putter or, if necessary, the putter and a wedge. Start by doing this for just a couple of holes and slowly build up your endurance over time. Be sure to wear your pedometer. Eventually you'll work your way up to walking a full nine holes – or maybe even 18 holes.

How much is enough? Again, to see improvements in blood pressure, you'd only need to take a moderate to brisk walk for 30 minutes or so three times a week. To achieve weight loss or to maintain your weight, increase that to five or six days weekly. To gain the most benefit for your health in general and your heart in particular, your goal would be to walk about 14 miles a week or the equivalent level in another physical activity.

Remember to make yourself that promise: stick with a programme of increased physical activity for just 90 days. If you do that you'll feel better and sleep better, and you'll never want to quit!

Energy requirements of common activities in METs

1 MET (metabolic equivalent) equals the amount of energy needed when the body is at rest.

- Sleeping
- Lying in bed
- Sitting quietly in a chair

2 METs equals twice the amount of energy used when at rest.

- Standing
- Talking
- Walking (1 mph)
- Reading
- Writing
- Playing cards
- Light housekeeping (dusting)
- Typing/word processing
- Shaving
- Dressing/brushing hair

2–3 METs

- Walking (2 mph)
- Playing piano
- Playing golf (electric cart)
- Bathing/showering
- Washing hair
- Moderate housework (light laundry)
- Preparing a meal
- Cycling (5 mph)
- Ten-pin bowling

3–4 METs

- Walking (3 mph)
- Cycling (8 mph)
- Driving in light traffic
- Climbing stairs slowly
- Heavier housework (scrubbing dishes)
- Ballroom dancing (foxtrot)
- Factory work

4–5 METs

- Walking (4 mph)
- Cycling (8 mph)
- Playing badminton/light tennis
- Heavy housework (mopping, vacuuming)

- Gardening/raking
- Light carpentry
- Mowing lawn (power)

- House painting
- Driving in heavy traffic
- Washing windows

5–6 METs

- Walking (4.5 mph)

- Golfing (carrying/pulling clubs)

- Cycling (10 mph)

- Very heavy housework (scrubbing floors)

- Roller-skating
- Light shovelling, digging

- Carrying wood or groceries
- Social dancing (tango)

6–7 METs

- Walking (5 mph)
- Cycling (11mph)
- Playing tennis (singles)
- Water-skiing
- Leisurely swimming

- Mowing lawn (hand mower)
- Square dancing
- Chopping wood
- Shovelling snow
- Moving furniture

7–8 METs

- Jogging (5 mph)
- Cycling (12 mph)
- Downhill skiing
- Canoeing
- Swimming lengths (slow)

- Playing football
- Horse riding at the gallop
- Climbing hills (moderate)
- Climbing stairs (continuous)
- Playing tennis (competitive singles)

8–9 METs

- Jogging (5.5 mph)
- Cycling (13 mph)
- Swimming lengths (fast)

- Cross-country skiing
- Playing basketball
- Carrying groceries upstairs

10+ METs

- Racquetball, squash
- Climbing hills with a load

- Jogging (6 mph and faster)

Chapter 7

The Mind/Body Connection

Not too many years ago, doctors dismissed the idea that mental health and physical health are inextricably linked. They were particularly condescending towards women, who learned to keep their feelings to themselves. The word 'hysteria' comes from the Greek word for womb ('*hustera*'), and has the connotation of acting emotionally, irrationally 'like a woman'. But the reality is that both men and women are, indeed, affected by their emotions, both positively and negatively.

I've seen how stress can have a horrible impact on cardiovascular health on many occasions, and I'm sure you have too. Have you ever said something like, 'This job is killing me', 'That wife/husband of mine is going to give me a heart attack', or 'Rush hour traffic makes my blood pressure sky-rocket'? Of course you have. We all have, so you are in good company.

Stress is like the weather. Everybody talks about it, but few do anything about it. Well, if it's raining, we can't wave a magic wand to make the sun shine, but we can open the umbrella to keep from getting soaked. We might get a bit wet, but we won't be drenched. And none of us would want to admit that we're 'too dumb to come in out of the rain'.

On the coming pages, I'd like to share some very personal observations, some solid scientific proof of the link between emotional states and blood pressure and heart attacks and strokes, and some suggestions that, yes, you can come in out of the emotional rain – or at least open that protective umbrella.

Why has the medical community not paid more attention to the mind/body connection? Part of it comes down to the lack of training in medical schools. And I think one major reason that negative emotional states aren't listed along with more traditional risk factors such as raised cholesterol levels and overweight and blood pressure is the inability to measure stress, depression, anger, hostility and anxiety directly and quantify those feelings in nice, discrete numbers on the patient's chart.

Fortunately, things seem to be changing. More and more doctors are starting to ask patients about their stress levels, especially when taking medical histories. And they're less likely today to state directly or imply that 'it's all in your mind' when counselling men and women. Medical schools are teaching about the mind/body connection. Typically, they've come up with a new word to legitimise the emerging new field: psycho-neurophysiology. That's a big word that just describes the link between the mind, the nervous system, and the many ways the body works.

Let me start with a few personal observations. I mentioned earlier that my father had severe hypertension and died of a heart attack. Or it might have been a stroke, since no autopsy was ever performed. One way or the other, there's no doubt in my mind that Dad's fatal cardiovascular event that terrible day in December 1969 was precipitated by overwhelming stress.

My father had been one of those lucky guys who really loved his work as a neighbourhood pharmacist. He was dearly beloved by his customers and he loved them back. Although he put in long hours in the store, he never really thought about it as 'work' in a negative way. Until a robbery at the pharmacy resulted in the savage stabbing of his assistant pharmacist, a man who was like a brother to him for many,

many years. Although Vince survived the attack, Dad's feelings about the store changed dramatically. Every time he opened the door in the morning, he was filled with dread at having to be at the scene of the crime.

In a matter of months, his health deteriorated and he visibly aged. My mother, brother and I, along with others, tried to convince Dad to simply get out of that store, fearing it would literally kill him. And it did. Whether it was a heart attack or a stroke doesn't matter. Dad had underlying cardiovascular disease and hypertension, and the stress was the precipitating factor that led to his death. I still miss him horribly.

And in my own case, in 1978 I was under overwhelming stress caused by a personal problem that I found impossible to resolve. I couldn't get it out of my mind. In retrospect, I think my blood pressure was probably sky-rocketing. And there were factors that had led to my underlying heart disease, including too many years of smoking two packs of cigarettes a day, living a mostly sedentary existence, and eating a diet high in saturated fat and cholesterol. I was unable to talk to anyone about my problems. I kept my fears and anxiety bottled up and the pressure built up to that day in May nearly three decades ago when I had my heart attack. I was lucky. Unlike my dad, I survived.

Next there's my own brother. Tom had always been a happy-go-lucky guy who liked his work and was so good at it that he didn't have to spend much time working to earn his very nice salary. Then his luck ran out. Financial woes became overwhelming and were always on his mind. It wasn't much of a surprise when he called from the hospital telling me that he had had a heart attack.

I've read case histories in the medical literature detailing how business executives in the cardiac care unit of the hospital where they were recovering from heart attacks confided that in a perverse way they were happy. Why? Because being in the hospital with no access to a telephone and with no visitors other than immediate family meant the first 'vacation' they'd had in years and the first time they were relieved of the responsibilities that led to a malignant level of stress.

And then there was a friend of mine, a maths teacher in middle school, working with children aged 11 to 13 years old. On the golf course at weekends, he'd tell me that, while he loved his work and loved the lasting impact he knew he was making on those boys and girls, he found the pressures and time constraints to be onerous. Fast forward: Chris suffered what turned out to be, not one, but three, simultaneous strokes. Happily, he survived, but the ill effects of that event forced him to take early retirement owing to disability.

Hey, I'm not trying to scare you. That's not my style. Rather, I'm trying to impress upon you just how important a role your emotional health plays on your cardiovascular health. If anything I've said thus far has made an impression, has reminded you of yourself, then you're now ready to learn just how the mind/body connection can lead to hypertension and what you can do to stop or at least slow down the insidious process.

It's rather ironic that our language is replete with terms and phrases including 'heart ache', 'heart break', 'heartfelt remark', 'heartless behaviour', 'be still my beating heart' and so on. We intuitively know that the heart is more than a chunk of muscle that pumps blood. The Japanese have an even more chilling term: *karoshi*. It means death from overwork.

The World Health Organization (WHO) Global Burden of Disease Survey estimates that by the year 2020 major depression will be second only to ischaemic heart disease in the degree of disability it will bring to those suffering from severely negative emotions. We're polluting our planet's earth, air and water. And we're polluting our bodies with stress, anxiety, anger, hostility and depression.

Job stress and blood pressure

It'll come as no surprise to anyone who dislikes his job or feels a lot of stress at work that most heart attacks occur on a Monday. Stress, it turns out, is, indeed, a killer. That's especially true when one's job expects high levels of performance but offers little in the way of control.

Investigators at University College London evaluated data from more than 10,000 civil service workers. Compared with subjects who didn't report job-related stress, those who told of work stress three or more times over the span of the 14-year study had double the risk of metabolic syndrome, which includes raised blood pressure along with other heart-related risk factors. Those complaining of work stress were typically in jobs with high expectations and low levels of control.

To better understand who is at risk, let's consider the lucky people who are not. Orchestral conductors tend to live long lives and continue their careers well after most people would want to retire. Why? They love their work, are truly passionate about their art, and despite potential frustration when the violinist or cello player doesn't hit a note just right, they have enormous control over their situation. Conductors are absolute bosses. Some might even call them tyrants.

On a lighter note, consider entertainers such as Bob Hope and many others who live well into their nineties. They, too, seldom retire. They enjoy their work and that work gives meaning to their lives. And why not? No one tells them what to do or when to do it. Sure, such men and women place high demands on themselves, but they are in control of their lives and their careers.

In the business world, the same can be said for top management. The highest-level executives make decisions and tell others to carry them out. Ultimately the real work falls on the shoulders of a low-echelon person who carries a large burden, never seems to catch up with the day's work, and has no control over how that work is to be done. He or she goes home each night thinking about the work still on the desk and knowing that tomorrow there will be even more.

Now let's intensify that scenario. The trip back home is not an idyllic ride through a beautiful valley filled with flowering shrubs and fluttering birds. No, it's more a matter of bumper-to-bumper traffic with knuckles white on the steering wheel. After 30, 40 or more minutes of near collisions and road rage, our worker finally comes home.

Forget the tableaus of 1950s-style television. Instead, there are crying children, appliances that have broken down, bills to pay, and a spouse whose day has been just as trying.

Doctors don't really understand why but, traditionally, women tended to be able to endure stress more successfully than men. It was the men whose blood pressure would just go up and up. But, sadly, that's changing. Now that women are trying to balance careers with the demands of raising children and managing the household, often with little or no help from their partners, they, too, are becoming hypertensive. Surely that's not what campaigners seeking equal opportunities for women had in mind?

Want to know the worst possible scenario? Combine job strain with poor home relationships, and you have the formula for sending your blood pressure through the roof. That was the conclusion of researchers at the University of Toronto, in Canada. They found that the amount of support given at home in a relationship is critical to health.

Because we live at a time when men and women must both work or at least both want to work, outside the home, we have to learn how to survive the situation. That means taking a bit of time, ideally away from the children, to actually talk. Ask about your spouse's day. Give him or her the chance to vent his or her frustrations.

Does that sound completely unrealistic? It can be done. It's a matter of realising the importance of relying on one another.

Here's my suggestion. At a time when things aren't at their very worst, when both of you are relatively at ease, think about setting a time each day to sit down for as little as ten minutes to just talk. And listen. Come on now, be honest with yourself. You find the time to spend hours and hours each week staring at the TV. Can't you assign ten minutes a day to improve your relationship and at the same time vent the emotions that can lead to hypertension?

Here's the reality. Job strain raises blood pressure during working hours. At first the body (notably your arteries) is quite resilient. When the whistle blows and it's time to quit for the day, blood pressure returns to normal. But when increases in blood pressure occur day after day, week after week, that resiliency diminishes and blood pressure eventually fails to return to normal. Picture your arteries as rubber bands that are repeatedly stretched to their limits. At some point the elasticity is gone and the rubber band breaks.

The 'type-A' personality and beyond

Two doctors in San Francisco, California, in the 1970s revolutionised the field of cardiology and added a term to the vocabulary worldwide. They described people who were angry, time-obsessed, and driven as having the 'type-A' personality. Those people were said to be at greater risk of developing heart disease and hypertension and of having heart attacks and strokes. But there was always something wrong with that picture.

If everyone who is driven by their career aspirations and by the need for success has a heart attack or stroke, how can we have successful businessmen, doctors, entertainers and world leaders? And how is it that the most successful of those actually live quite long lives? And if some people aren't obsessed with time and deadlines, newspapers could never hit the stands – and this book would never have been written!

It turns out that the concept of the type-A personality had it only half right. It's the anger and hostility that can develop out of stressful situations, especially in those prone to such negative emotions, that kills. A long-term study of more than 1,000 men found that those who had angry or irritable responses to stressful situations were three times more likely to be diagnosed with heart disease and five times more likely to suffer a heart attack before the age of 55. Another investigation showed that women with heart disease who were hostile had double the risk of having a heart attack or dying from heart problems than women who weren't hostile.

Most times the process is slow and insidious. Hypertension, and resultant heart attacks and strokes, doesn't develop overnight. But in our stress-ridden society anger and hostility can kill suddenly and dramatically. It was a California psychologist who coined the term 'road rage' to describe the behaviour displayed when too many cars clog that state's roads and freeways. It sounds absurd, but this scenario has been played out too many times: one driver is cut up by another guy, he flashes an obscene gesture in anger, and the other driver gets out and starts a fight. And it's not just men. I've seen women screaming at each other over a contested parking place in a shopping mall.

Exaggerated examples? Such behaviour occurs every day. Going back to the worker with huge job demands and little control, we now have the term 'going postal' to describe the sometimes fatal anger and fury that can boil over. That term was coined when post office workers 'solved' their problems with blazing guns.

Every country has its problems. A Japanese study classified workers by the amount of overtime put in. Investigators found that while there were no significant differences in conventionally measured blood pressures, those who worked an average of 60 extra hours or more a month had higher 24-hour blood pressure levels. Both BP and heart rate were higher when workers were accumulating overtime.

In England, a study was conducted with 10,000 civil servants. Those in the lowest grades of the administration were at the highest risk for cardiovascular diseases. During work hours, blood pressure went up. And the lower the person was on the administrative ladder the higher the pressure went.

As human beings, we're not the only creatures who respond very badly to stress. Hans Selye, a Canadian researcher credited with being a pioneer of stress research, used ordinary house mice as his test subjects. As his mouse population grew in a confined space, males fought more aggressively over territory, sometimes to the death. And females ceased to reproduce.

How emotions kill

Stress and other negative emotions affect our bodies in very tangible, physiological ways. As one example, especially for those who are prone to irregular heart rhythms (arrhythmias), mental stress can trigger dangerous disruptions in heartbeat. Those disruptions can be enough to cause a heart attack. But even those without existing arrhythmias can be at risk, as has been tragically demonstrated at such disasters as the World Trade Center attack in New York. Following that attack, cardiovascular events including heart attacks and strokes multiplied.

Mental stress can trigger a lack of blood flow to the heart, thus increasing the risk of death in people with already clogged arteries. Such mental stress increases oxygen demand because blood pressure and heart rate go up. At the same time, stiffened arteries resist increased blood flow and coronary arteries in the heart constrict, further decreasing blood supply.

Mental stress also causes the inner layer of the blood vessels to constrict, which may increase the risk of sudden cardiac death. Sudden stress leads to 'endothelial dysfunction', the medical term for malfunction of those arterial linings when the artery's ability to dilate is impaired. Swiss researchers found a significant decrease in blood vessel dilation after mental stress. Diastolic blood pressure shot up from 83 to 96 and heart rate rose from 63 to 81 beats per minute.

Doctors can actually measure the chemicals that rush into your bloodstream during stress, anger and hostility. Cortisol, adrenaline, noradrenaline and others not worth memorising or even hearing all raise blood pressure. Since early in our evolution, those chemicals have prepared us for fight or flight. Cavemen, I'm sure, experienced tremendous anxiety when they encountered vicious animals intent on turning them into dinner. But once the fight or flight was over, those early men leaned against a rock or a tree and relaxed. Later they might have bragged about their victory while sitting around the fire. But their stress was not relentless. That's a curse of modern times for too many men and women.

Hypertensive men who don't manage stressful situations well may be at increased risk of stroke, according to doctors working in Sweden. Those researchers monitored 238 hypertensive men between 1982 and 1996. They concluded that those who fail to find successful strategies to manage a situation or solve a conflict are in most trouble. Such individuals don't work methodically. They try a number of strategies without giving them enough time to see if they work. In the long run, that kind of behaviour creates wear and tear on the body.

Let's look at it in a step-by-step fashion. You find yourself under mental stress at work, but don't find a way to cope with that stress. Blood pressure goes up during those working hours. The stressful situation is repeated daily. At first BP returns to normal when the work whistle blows. Eventually BP remains raised even during non-working hours. Now you're formally hypertensive. As a hypertensive patient, you are now more at risk of heart attack or stroke when faced with a sudden, intense emotion of whatever sort. That risk is, of course, multiplied many times by a concurrent rise in cholesterol, sedentary lifestyle, cigarette smoking, diabetes and other factors. That's not a good crystal ball to gaze into, is it?

Some still contend that work-related or other forms of stress play no significant role. I find it difficult to say that hostility and anger and anxiety have no effect on the development of hypertension and cardiovascular disease when one can simply strap on a blood pressure cuff and see what happens when one starts thinking of whatever it is in one's life that might cause such hostility, anger and anxiety. Again, you can make your own decision as to whether this is an area that's worth your while to deal with in your life.

Learn to control your stress

You have a tremendous ability to control the mind/body connection. It takes no special talent, and you don't have to become a meditating monk living far from the pressures of civilisation. Here's one simple demonstration. Close your eyes for just a moment and think about a lemon. Picture yourself slicing that lemon and watching the juices flow. You can smell that lemony aroma. Now imagine picking up a slice and putting it into your mouth and sucking on the tart, juicy fruit.

What happened? Your mouth started to water. Unless you have some sort of underlying disorder that limits your ability to salivate, it's almost impossible not to have your mouth water when thinking about that juicy lemon. In a very real way, your mental thoughts have had a dramatic effect on your body.

The mind is a wonderful, awesome thing. Try not to think of elephants. Really. Put elephants completely out of your mind. When trying not to do so, you just can't seem to make those big creatures go away. And we've all had those times when we can't get the words or melody of a song out of our minds.

Here's an experiment to try when you get a home BP monitor, which I really hope you will do. Put the cuff around your arm and measure your pressure. Note the reading. Now think about something that happened in your life either recently or a while back that really made you angry. Dwell on that negative experience for two or three minutes. Then measure your BP again. Almost certainly the numbers will be higher.

The good news is that you can do exactly the opposite, whether you're hooked up to a monitor or not. It might sound strange, but thinking 'happy thoughts' at times when a situation would normally generate anger or hostility can 'medicate' your mind. Pleasant thoughts cause the release of relaxing neurotransmitters in the brain. This is not wishful thinking, but rather a scientific fact that has been documented by high-tech brain scans, showing the very positive effects of such mental manipulations.

As with any other endeavour, learning to cope with stress takes some effort and your ability will increase with practice. The following coping suggestions can have a very real, physical effect on your brain and your emotional status. And they can help control blood pressure, just as surely as prescription anti-anxiety medications can do. Both increase levels of serotonin, 'the happy neurotransmitter', in the brain.

I've proved this time and time again with friends and relatives who were having an attack of hiccups. Hiccups, you ask? What do hiccups have to do with blood pressure? Well, nothing, really. But what I'm about to describe is a fairly dramatic demonstration of just how well one can control one's bodily functions.

Hiccups are caused by spasms of the diaphragm that are followed by sudden closing of the glottis at the back of the throat, interrupting air flow and resulting in the characteristic 'hiccup' sound. Hiccups follow irritation of nerves that control the respiratory muscles, particularly the diaphragm. Many things, from swallowing hot or irritating foods or drinks to bouts of joyous laughter, can cause them. We've all heard of this cure or that: holding one's breath, putting a paper bag over the head, being startled. Sometimes they work, most times they don't. But my cure is, trust me, 100 per cent effective each and every time.

And it demonstrates how you can, indeed, affect a malfunctioning part of the body. You can, in this case, stop the spasms of the diaphragm and, *voila*, the hiccups are gone. So, here we go. And, please, don't roll your eyes or think this is in the realm of weirdo-hippy gobbledegook. Try this technique the next time you or someone else gets those hiccups.

Find a place where you can be alone. You can't concentrate effectively if you're with other people – even just a couple. Ideally, turn the lights down, not necessarily off. Sit with your back straight and your legs crossed with your arms on top of your legs with palms up and fingers gently bent. Yeah, I know, you're already starting to think Indian guru nonsense. Again, bear with me. Don't knock it till you've tried it.

Close your eyes. Take a deep, deep breath and think of your chest as a balloon that's filling to maximum capacity. When you think you've taken in as much air as you can hold, 'sip' in a little more. Then hold your breath as long as you can, with your back still straight. Now slowly, slowly release your breath. As you do so, imagine your body is a balloon that has a puncture and the air is gradually leaking out, causing the balloon to deflate. As you exhale, allow your body to fall forwards, chest towards your legs. At the point when you think all the air is exhaled, 'puff' a couple more breaths out.

Then very slowly begin to breathe air back into that 'balloon', inflating it as your back returns to the upright position. Think about that air. Feel how your body inflates and then deflates. Do that a few times. Feel yourself totally relaxing. You're thinking about nothing but your breathing in and out, in and out. And then, bingo!, your hiccups will be gone.

This technique has never failed. And everyone I've ever showed it to has become a zealot, teaching others how to do it. Try it the next time you get hiccups.

You'll find that you get an unexpected bonus. You'll wind

up feeling remarkably relaxed. And that leads me into why I share this little tip with you. You don't have to wait for hiccups to get that relaxed feeling. You can do this little routine every day. And, indeed, you should do so. The more often you try it, the better you'll get at achieving a remarkable state of relaxation.

With a bit of practice, you'll find that just as you're able to stop a bout of hiccups, you can stop an episode of anxiety. But don't wait for an anxious, stressful moment. As with any other skill, this one takes some practice. So do your practising when you're not anxious or upset or angry. I like to think of it as taking a mini-holiday during the day. No matter where you are – at work, at home or elsewhere – you can find a quiet place to gain a sense of peace.

If you wait until you're in a bad mood, without first practising the technique, you'll be too upset to achieve self-soothing. If you've done it a number of times before you really need to, you'll find that you can breathe your anger away. Really and truly.

Even if you're sitting at a conference table with business associates – or family members for that matter – you can at least do some deep breathing. Remember that old saw, 'Count to ten before losing your temper'? Try taking ten deep, deep breaths in and out, thinking about your breathing, to relieve some of your anxiety.

As time goes on, you very well may come to appreciate the soothing feeling you can achieve with that kind of breathing. You might graduate to taking five or ten minutes once or twice a day to simply take one of those mini-holidays. What you're doing is a sort of meditation. And while you might baulk at the very word 'meditation', isn't meditation better and more preferable to medication?

You might also want to try what's called 'mindfulness'. Unlike the sort of meditation that most people are, if not familiar with, at least aware of, mindfulness is a conscious effort to think or to concentrate. In meditation, people try to clear their minds of all thought. And that's not everyone's cup of tea. It's surely not mine. I prefer to be mindful of, say, my breathing. Or, while taking a walk, I'll concentrate and really think about the mechanics of walking: striding forward while balancing on the back leg, then flexing the back foot and pushing that leg forward as the other leg moves to the back, and so forth. Or think about your heart beating in your chest and how it's pumping blood through the miles of arteries to every nook and cranny of your body. Or look into the sky and marvel at the clouds. You can do this even while you're working at home or at some task – unless you're operating a chain saw or a factory press, of course!

Psychologists have developed a technique called biofeedback, in which one concentrates on heartbeat or breathing. The feedback comes from a machine that registers blood pressure or heart rate or both. The apparatus and training can be expensive, but some find biofeedback to be very helpful.

There's a far less expensive tool I can recommend that helps you become effective at relaxing your breathing. It's called RESPeRATE, a device that runs you through breathing exercises and has been clinically proven to be beneficial in controlling both stress and hypertension (see also pages 194–5). You can learn more about RESPeRATE and order it online at www.high-blood-pressure-help.com.

What are some other ways of coping with stress?

Virtually all doctors and psychologists agree that one of the best is exercise (see page 78). If 'exercise' is a dirty word to you, think of it as merely physical activity. In other words, you don't have to go to a gym and run endlessly on a treadmill. Relaxing physical activity can be anything you enjoy doing. Studies comparing the 'mechanics' of various activities have shown that one can achieve similar 'work' when gardening, dancing, cycling, walking in the woods, opting to walk the golf course rather than use a golf cart, or even cleaning the house at a brisk pace. My wife has learned that when I get angry about something, I tend to clean the kitchen or do some other chore at nearly break-neck pace. Of course, she doesn't mind a bit!

Then there's 'work' versus work. One man's work is another man's pleasure or hobby as it were. Probably the last thing a professional carpenter would want to do in his spare time is woodwork. But for a number of men I've known, who make their living in a law court, business office or hospital, woodwork in the basement, perhaps making a nest box, is an absolute joy. Try putting together a jigsaw puzzle. Or get a pair of binoculars and a bird book to identify the birds in your garden. Whatever the hobby might be, find something you can enjoy to take your mind off things that cause stress.

By the way, watching TV is not a good way to relax. Without going into unnecessary technical details, the brain does not relax when gazing at the screen in the same way it might when solving a crossword puzzle or reading a book or magazine. Limit the time you spend in front of the tube and expand your activities to other things.

Are you an animal lover? Many studies have confirmed that stroking a dog or taking it for a walk makes the blood pressure plummet. Some doctors and psychologists have gone so far as to strongly recommend that patients get a pet. And many care facilities for the elderly have taken in dogs and cats to help residents stay relaxed.

Here's something to really think about. Are you nice to yourself? How well do you treat yourself? Most men and women do far more for others than they do for themselves, and make themselves the lowest priority. Do something nice for yourself, not just once in a while but on a regular basis. My wife really likes to have a facial. I prefer a massage, which I schedule on late Friday afternoons every two weeks. It's something I look forward to, and a nice way to end the working week and start the weekend on a relaxing note. Too expensive? There are massage schools that offer cut-rate services from students. On Sunday mornings, my wife loves to make herself a bowl of porridge and do a crossword puzzle while eating it, no matter how much work she has waiting to do that day. And at weekends you'll seldom find me in the office. I'll be out rambling or playing golf or fishing with some friends. While I'm doing one of those things, my wife will be playing a game of duplicate bridge; she's a life master and takes the game quite seriously. Both my wife and I work very hard, putting in long hours every week, but we both make sure there's time for fun and games! We deserve it, and so do you.

Five words to live by

The next time you find yourself steaming with anger over something, ask yourself this simple, five-word question: **Is it worth dying for?** There's no doubt in my mind that if my father knew that the stress he was experiencing in the months before his death would lead to that fatal heart attack or stroke, he would have locked the store and never gone back. He could have eventually sold the pharmacy and made a decent living as a pharmacist working elsewhere.

Is work killing you? Either find a way to cope with that job or get a different one. Does your spouse make you angry far too often? Get marital counselling. Are there issues that have you losing sleep at night? Perhaps there's a friend or a clergyman you can confide in. Speak to your doctor about therapy or prescription drugs or both. The list could go on and on. Only you know your 'triggers'. And only you can seek a solution if the coping mechanisms I've suggested just aren't enough and if you know your blood pressure is going up. Take the pressure off your heart.

Keep those five words in mind: **Is it worth dying for?** You know that the answer is, of course, 'Hell, no!'

Chapter 8

No Butts About It: Time to Quit Smoking

You've heard all the statistics. It has been estimated that in the UK smoking kills more than 114,000 men and women every year – one-fifth of all deaths – mostly due to bronchitis, emphysema, lung cancer, heart disease and strokes. In the US that number is 400,000 deaths annually. A UK study calculated that the average smoker burns up £80,000 in a lifetime. Smoking bans in English and Irish pubs would have been unthinkable ten years ago, but today they are a reality. If you smoke, you very likely resent such intrusions into your rights and your life.

As a former smoker myself, I know just how you feel. And, believe me, right from the start, I'm not going to pontificate. I'm not going to try to convince you to quit. You've heard that from your doctor, your partner, boyfriend or girlfriend, your children, your friends. But if you're ready to quit, I'll help you do it. And I'll point to others who can give more assistance.

The reality is that those who successfully give up smoking really **want** to quit. They haven't been talked into it or frightened into it. They've finally hit the wall and truthfully said to themselves, 'I **want** to give up.' Just saying 'I should give up' won't do it. I hope you now want to stop smoking, just like I finally really wanted to 26 years ago when I finally said goodbye to my friend and lover, my cigarettes.

Non-smokers just don't understand smokers. 'Hey, it's just a habit, get over it!' 'Millions of other smokers have quit, so you can too.' 'If you really loved me, you'd quit.'

As one smoker said to me, during a coffee break at work when we were both puffing away, 'I can't imagine living without smoking.' I couldn't either. Smoking was part of my life. Hell, my cigarettes were my best friends. Only more dependable, to be there whenever I wanted to celebrate, commiserate or anything in between. More than just a friend, my cigarette was my lover. Paul Simon sang, 'There must be fifty ways to leave your lover,' but I hadn't found one that worked for me.

As Mark Twain once famously said, 'It's easy to quit, I've done it many times.' But until the time I finally stopped for good, my quitting never lasted more than a couple of days.

Trained as a journalist in college, I was forever in a cloud of blue smoke, my own and that of others. Coffee and cigarettes were our fuel. We couldn't imagine writing without both, especially the cigarettes. My brand was Marlboro, and when I was about 18 years old I actually thought about getting the Marlboro man's tattoo on the back of my hand just like his. It looked so 'cool' when he'd light his weed from a glowing stick he pulled out of the campfire in those TV ads of the 1960s. Hey, forget the fact that the Marlboro man died of lung cancer.

Even my professor in physiology during my graduate training was a smoker. He often smoked while giving his lectures. I learned years later that he died of a heart attack.

After graduating from college I had a terrific job, making quite a bit of money for a young guy. I couldn't pick up the phone without lighting a cigarette. Or attend a meeting. Or have a cup of coffee. I remember saying that I'd gladly write a cheque for $1,000 to someone who could give me an injection or a pill so I could wake up in the morning as a non-smoker. Those were the days when $1,000 was big money, by the way. But, I also said, I wouldn't take a cheque for $1,000 to quit, since I knew I couldn't.

Did you 'practise' smoking in front of a mirror when you first started to smoke? I did. I learned to 'French inhale' the smoke into my nostrils from my mouth. I tried to look like European actors I'd seen in the movies. And I loved playing with my Zippo lighter. I loved it!

The day I came home to my apartment after being discharged from the hospital in 1978 after my first bypass surgery, I made a martini and lit a Marlboro. After all, my surgeon told me I had had something wrong and he fixed it. He said to enjoy my life and forget all about the surgery. Later on, my cardiologist, an internationally renowned man, said that the six or so cigarettes I smoked during the day (I had coincidentally cut down during that time) probably weren't too bad if they helped me to relax at the end of the day. The medical consensus has changed since then!

I quit one day in July in 1979. By that time I not only knew I should quit, I really wanted to quit. I didn't *choose* to smoke those 40 cigarettes a day, I *had* to. They were controlling me, I wasn't controlling them. It was impossible for me to smoke only those cigarettes that I actually enjoyed. Getting deathly ill was my lucky break. I woke up one morning with a horrible sore throat. I tried to inhale my first cigarette of the day and the smoke felt like razor blades. So I thought that I wouldn't smoke for the rest of the day. In fact, I put the last of my pack in the bin. The next morning, still sick as a dog, I went out and bought another pack. I lit one and it was just as bad. Okay, I said, one more day without smoking. And I threw the pack away and went back up to the apartment and into bed. That went on for almost a week. Then I thought, hey, this is the longest I've ever gone without a smoke. I wondered if I could just do 'one more day'.

Like an alcoholic who's gone to Alcoholics Anonymous, I lived my life going 'one more day' without smoking for the next few weeks. Back at work, I chewed a toothpick or sucked boiled sweets at meetings. And I adopted quite a few tricks and techniques to help me live my life without cigarettes. Was it tough? Probably the most difficult thing I've ever done. Did it work? I've been a non-smoker since that day in July in 1979.

In this chapter I'm going to share with you some of the tips that helped me to succeed. And I'll detail the information I've gained by doing research with major health groups, compare methods of quitting, and examine some of the aids that didn't exist back in 1979. If you've finally come to that time in your life when you **want** to stop smoking, when you're literally sick and tired of smoking, and when you finally admit to yourself that you no longer smoke for pleasure, you smoke because you **have** to smoke, and that you down deep inside **hate** those cigarettes as much or more than you love them, I know I can help.

When not to quit

In an ideal world, anytime would be a good time to stop smoking. But we live in a real world. Don't try to do it when you're under an exceptional amount of stress, because you're likely to fail, and that'll just convince you that you can't quit. If you were served with divorce papers today, it might not be the best time to give up cigarettes. So you might think that going on holiday would be a great time to leave the cigarettes behind. But the harsh facts are that you'll be edgy, irritable, and miserable and make those around you unhappy as well. Don't spoil that holiday.

Instead, pick a day like any other day. A typical day, nothing unusual. Hey, we're all under a certain amount of stress at work and at home, so you can't expect to have a stress-free day that would be the idyllic time to stop smoking. And even if you did, that wouldn't necessarily prepare you for ordinary days.

Many support groups suggest picking a day on the calendar some time in the future. Some day next week or next month. Start preparing for your 'quit date' by stocking up on stuff to keep your mind off the cigarettes and things to 'play' with to keep your hands occupied. Lay in a supply of toothpicks, hardboiled sweets, chewing gum, bottled water, worry beads, nicotine patches and healthy snacks. Tell all your friends and family in advance. The problem with planning is that you might postpone that 'quit date' and wind up feeling so embarrassed that it'll discourage you from future attempts. But many people have, indeed, used that planning technique successfully.

A British study indicates that the best approach might be simply to decide one day, that's it, I'm giving up smoking. And just do it. Starting that day. No putting it off any more. That's like jumping right into a pool of cold water rather than starting by dipping in a toe, and then a foot, and so on. In retrospect, that's just what I did. I woke up sick, the cigarette hurt my throat, and I decided to quit. In the past I'd made bets with my college room-mates, promised a girlfriend that I'd quit, made plans to do so during the college recess or whatever. For me, at least, that never worked. In talking with fellow ex-smokers, the majority said they made a spontaneous decision one day and never smoked again.

Ultimately, it will be your decision as to when you quit, and how. In the meantime, let me point out the effect your next cigarette will have on your body. Smoking just one cigarette can cause a sudden change in how well your heart beats. Your blood pressure goes up. Your arteries constrict. These are not good things to happen. But let's look at some of the good things that you'll experience when you do stop smoking.

Benefits over time

Just 20 minutes after your last cigarette, your blood pressure starts to go down. Your heart rate slows. And your hands and feet start feeling warmer, demonstrating the almost immediate improvement in circulation. Within eight hours, carbon monoxide levels in your blood drop to normal, replaced by invigorating oxygen. By the end of the first day, in a mere 24 hours, your chances of suffering a heart attack or stroke go down. And after two smoke-free days your nerve endings return to normal function and your ability to smell and taste improves. A major consideration is reduced risk of emphysema and osteoporosis.

Over a period of time, from two weeks to three months, your circulation will improve significantly. Smokers tend to feel the cold more than non-smokers in the same temperatures. You'll find that walking and other exercise gets easier as your lung function improves. Sports coaches were among the first to urge athletes to quit, even before doctors, because they saw how smoking saps performance. Pay attention to those improvements in yourself and remind yourself that these are the rewards for the discomforts you've been feeling, because, let's face the facts, quitting isn't easy or pleasant. But I can tell you this: it's better than a heart attack. I've been there. I know.

In the coming months, you'll feel better and better. You'll cough less and less. Sinus congestion diminishes. You'll feel more energy and less fatigue. Notice when you climb a flight of stairs that you're not as short of breath.

By the end of the first non-smoking year, your risk of heart disease is down to half that of a smoker. After five to 15 years, the risk of your suffering a stroke is cut to the same level as those who have never smoked. When you celebrate your tenth anniversary of giving up smoking, remember that your risk of lung cancer is half that of smokers. You'll also improve your odds against a wide variety of other cancers – and ulcers, too.

In 15 years, your risk of heart disease is no different from men and women who never smoked a cigarette. Your expected life span will be about the same as well.

All those statistics were part of the US Surgeon General's report in 1990. I can add from personal experience and from what I've learned from others that you'll sleep better, wake up more rested, have more energy and just feel better in general.

Those nasty withdrawal symptoms

Why is it so difficult to give up? Smoking is far more than a bad habit, like squeezing the toothpaste in the middle of the tube. You have both a powerful psychological pattern and a true chemical addiction that are as strong as being hooked on heroin or cocaine. Non-smokers just don't understand that, and neither did the medical profession until fairly recently. Former heroin addicts have told me that quitting that drug was *easier* than giving up cigarettes.

Here's something to think about. A heavily addicted drug addict might 'shoot up' three or four times a day. If you smoke a pack a day, you're getting a 'fix' 20 times daily. I smoked two packets of Marlboros a day at my point of deepest addiction. So I needed *40 fixes each and every day*! Modern medical imaging systems allow scientists to look at the brain before and after either a 'hit' of drug or a 'puff' from a cigarette. The pictures look the same. In technical terms, dopamine receptor sites in the brain crave the next wave of satisfaction.

There is something that smokers do not realise. I know I didn't. To me, I looked forward to having the next cigarette. I said I enjoyed that cigarette. That was especially true when I had to go without a smoke for a longer than average time, such as at the cinema or in church. Ah… That cigarette I craved tasted so good! But the reality is very different from enjoying a fine piece of chocolate, or the scent of the Christmas tree when it first goes up in December.

In truth, you're not really enjoying the taste of the cigarette. You're enjoying the freedom from the craving that's been emanating from your brain and affecting your entire body. After having, say, that piece of chocolate, do you have a strong craving an hour or so later? I'm talking about a craving so demanding that you'd go to the waste bin to find the chocolate wrapper and lick it to get a little taste? Like the way I know you do when you're out of cigarettes in the middle of the night and you light up a cigarette stub from the ashtray? There's no comparison. Craving a cigarette is a demonstration of addiction, not appreciation.

The source of that addiction is nicotine. Try to switch to a low-tar cigarette and you'll simply smoke more to get the amount of nicotine you need. Not want, *need*. The tobacco companies have known that for decades and they've made sure that cigarettes deliver the amount of nicotine a smoker craves. Cigarettes truly are delivery systems for nicotine, a substance just as addictive as any other drug.

The bad news is that you'll start experiencing nicotine withdrawal symptoms at the exact moment when you'd normally light your next cigarette. The first of those symptoms will be edginess, restlessness, irritability and general frustration that might even make you prowl the room like a caged tiger. You might have trouble concentrating; that was particularly difficult for me at the typewriter. Some experience dizziness during the first day or two. Others go into a bit of depression, or might have trouble sleeping, or find themselves feeling hungry all the time. I'll talk about the weight issue a bit later.

At the beginning, there's only one way to get rid of all those symptoms instantly. Light another cigarette. Don't do it. The worst will come after two or three days of withdrawal. Then the cravings and withdrawal symptoms will gradually decrease. The good news is that, typically after just two or three weeks, your body is free of nicotine addiction. That is to say, those receptor sites in the brain will no longer be screaming at you to light another cigarette stub.

Now here's a radical concept. Instead of viewing those withdrawal symptoms as painful and horrible and of no value, make an active, conscious effort to accept each craving as a part of the learning curve. When the urge to light up becomes almost unbearable, *think* about how that craving will pass and how such desires are becoming fewer and further between. Moreover, think about that craving, though unquestionably painful, as a small price to pay for the freedom you're fighting for. That's right, you've become a freedom fighter, battling an addiction that has killed millions but that has been beaten by millions more. Notice that today you have had fewer cravings than yesterday. Tomorrow there will be fewer still. And you're able to deal with and beat back that craving more effectively with each passing day. If you're a religious person, by all means ask for divine assistance. Pray to get through that compelling desire. Or think intensively about the many reasons you want to quit. Work your way through each wave of craving by taking an active role: go for a walk for a few minutes, maybe this is the time to clean your shoes or empty the bin, do a few sit-ups, or whatever can take your mind off the moment. Remember always that the physical withdrawal symptoms will last, at most, only a few weeks.

Unfortunately, there is also the psychological addiction, far worse than the word 'habit' implies. The reason is very simple. We smokers learned to smoke a cigarette at any time – including when we're making a phone call, drinking a cup of coffee, or following lovemaking. Those associations are difficult to break. We literally have to learn *not* to smoke at each and every one of those cues. The more cigarettes one smokes during a typical day, over the course of a week or more, the greater the number of those cues.

While that may seem enormously difficult at first, it can help you find a way to break up the quitting process into manageable bites. First, decide what your most frequent, most urgent cues are. Yours will be different from mine. A college room-mate of mine always smoked a cigarette while sitting on the toilet in the morning. When he quit, that daily bowel movement brought the urge to light up. Spend a little time thinking about your strongest associations. Jot those times down on a piece of paper. Then think about what you can do to break those particular habits one at a time.

Here are a few suggestions:

- Instead of having a cup of coffee during the morning and afternoon break, go for a ten-minute walk.
- Rather than lingering at the dinner table after a meal, get up at once and start the washing-up.
- Replace your cigarette packet with a bag of bitter lemon sweets or mints for something to reach for when the phone rings or an office meeting begins. A barman I knew kept a pocketful of swizzle sticks to chew during the day.

As time goes on, and the cravings and desires pass, you'll be able to live through each and every one of those cues without both the cigarettes and their temporary replacements and diversions. But don't be surprised if, even months or years later, something signals an urge to light a cigarette.

I remember that one evening my wife, Dawn, and I were having a drink at one of the few bars in Los Angeles with a commanding view of the city. It's called the SkyBar. Seated at a table next to the floor-to-ceiling window and gazing out at the sparkling lights beneath us, I had this powerful desire to have a cigarette. That was about six years after I'd stopped smoking, and I thought the habit was completely broken. So what was going on?

In Chicago, where Dawn and I had lived before moving west to California, we enjoyed countless evenings in just such a setting. We were both smokers at the time. The pleasures of those evenings and smoking were strongly linked. It had been years since those days of high-rise apartments, restaurants and bars in the 'Windy City'. That view from the SkyBar window sparked those memories and those cravings for a cigarette. I had not yet learned to enjoy such moments without lighting up. So that evening I did just that. In a few minutes, the craving was gone and Dawn and I had a good laugh over it. And I never again experienced that craving in similar circumstances.

When I quit, I took being a non-smoker one day at a time. I recommend that you do the same. Don't try to imagine not smoking for the rest of your life. That's too much to take at once.

As each day went by, the craving became less persistent. A few techniques definitely helped. For example:

- Getting up from a chair and walking across the room.
- Taking a deep breath, and concentrating on breathing to take my mind off the craving.
- Having a sip of water.
- Playing a game of solitaire to keep my hands busy.
- Going to the cinema, theatre or anywhere else that smoking was prohibited.

Smoking cessation aids

Although the psychological addiction takes longer to deal with, it isn't as dramatic or as traumatic as withdrawal from nicotine. Fortunately there are several aids to help wean smokers off nicotine gradually. They work better for some people than for others. But you owe it to yourself to give them a try to improve your chances of success. While many people quit without using those aids, people who give in and light up again do so primarily because of the strength of that nicotine addiction and craving.

Nicotine replacement by way of patches, gum, lozenges, inhalers and sprays is a way of tapering off the amount of nicotine your body needs on a daily basis to maintain a sense of 'equilibrium' and comfort. These aids greatly reduce withdrawal symptoms. Pregnant women and those with existing heart disease should speak to a doctor before using nicotine replacement.

Studies have shown that nicotine replacement greatly improves one's chances of quitting successfully. And combining that with a support group of some kind can double the chances of success. More about those support groups later.

If you're going to use a smoking cessation aid, it's best to do so from the very start, rather than waiting until the withdrawal symptoms are becoming intolerable. You need all the help you can get. I wish those aids had been around in 1979!

For details concerning the various nicotine replacement aids, including how best to use them and potential side effects, visit the website www.cancer.org or one of the other sources of information I've provided at the end of this chapter. You may also want to discuss their use with your doctor.

Prescription drugs

Virtually everyone who stops smoking goes through a period of significant stress. Irritability, restlessness, inability to concentrate on one's work and other symptoms are pretty common. Adding this to one's everyday stress and strains may undermine success in giving up.

The drug bupropion hydrochloride (Zyban) is a prescription-only anti-depressant that has been successfully used to help smokers stop. However, this drug can raise blood pressure (see pages 208–9). Again, talk to your doctor about possibly getting a prescription to help cope with the emotional effects of giving up smoking.

In addition to those drugs, there are other ways of dealing with stress, both while attempting to stop smoking and at other times as well. Regular exercise is one of the best coping tools (see page 78). Rigorous physical activity, in fact, causes the brain to release the body's natural relaxants, the beta-endorphins, that can have a truly potent soothing effect. Many of us who are 'hooked' on exercise really enjoy the feeling that a good workout can provide. And the effects last for hours, well into the day or evening. For more approaches to stress control, see Chapter 7: The Mind/Body Connection.

Support groups and other aids

The best support while trying to stop smoking should come from one's family, friends and colleagues at work. When you decide to quit, tell them all. Many will be former smokers, familiar with the difficulties of giving up smoking. They'll remember how they were grumpy and irritable themselves during the withdrawal period. Explain to those who have never smoked that your grouchiness and occasional nastiness has nothing to do with them, and ask them to be as under-standing as possible.

In addition, there are both non-profit and for-profit organisations that can help you get over this hurdle in your life. The best of these groups will include either individual or group counselling. Choose a support group that offers in-depth assistance in terms of offering more or longer sessions, or both. There are definite similarities here with alcoholic treatment centres. In fact, one group is called Nicotine Anonymous. You'll want to have sessions at least 20 to 30 minutes long each time, frequently throughout the week, for at least two to three weeks.

'Together' is a free programme provided by the NHS Stop smoking support team. For details, call the NHS Smoking Helpline on 0800 169 0 169 or visit the website:

www.givingupsmoking.co.uk. Many GP surgeries, health clinics and hospitals run local stop smoking support groups. Your doctor will have details.

Other smoking cessation services include QUIT, an independent charity that helps smokers to stop. It also runs specialist smoking cessation services for pregnant smokers and their partners and Asian people. The Quitline, 0800 002 200, is open until 9pm, seven days a week.

Hypnosis and acupuncture are controversial methods to help smokers give up cigarettes. Some health authorities feel that there is no scientific evidence that either really works. Others see potential benefits and recommend that smokers give them a try. Certainly one can find non-smokers who swear by one or other method. If you've tried to give up again and again without success, you might want to give one or both a try.

Weight gain

Decades ago, tobacco companies advertised their deadly products as a way to lose and maintain weight. Indeed, the sad fact is that those who quit smoking often do gain weight. That's more the case for women than for men, though both are likely to put on a few pounds while shedding the cigarette habit.

Don't let the prospect of weight gain deter you from your resolve to stop smoking cigarettes. Certainly the health benefits of quitting far outbalance the ill effects of slight weight gain. And once you're comfortable in your life as a non-smoker, you can deal with getting rid of the weight you put on during that life-saving effort.

But there are definitely ways you can, at the very least, limit the amount of weight you will gain. Follow a healthy diet that's low in fat, nutrient-poor carbohydrates and calories. When choosing snacks and 'nibbles' to replace cigarettes throughout the day, opt for those lowest in calories such as pretzels, popcorn, sugar-free sweets, carrot sticks, celery stalks and the like. And be certain to engage in some physical activity each and every day.

Quid pro quo

That's a term often used in the practice of law to indicate a trade off, literally translated as 'this for that'. Offer yourself a reward for giving up cigarettes. Work out how much money you spend on smoking each day, week, month and year. You'll probably be shocked at the large figure you come up with even though you're already aware that it's been an expensive habit. Then decide what you'd rather do with the money you'll save.

Start a 'quitter's bank' and put the money you've saved each week in a coffee tin or pickle jar. Keep that money out of your ordinary budget for necessities. Maybe you'll have enough to buy a piece of jewellery. Or perhaps you'd prefer a long weekend with your partner or a friend. It's your choice, and you deserve it!

Helping a smoker quit

If your friend or loved one has decided to give up smoking, you can and will play an important role in his or her success or failure. You might, for example, be tempted to tell that person to light up a cigarette just to end the grumpiness. That's happened more than once in lots and lots of families. That's not a good idea. Similarly, you don't want to tell him or her how to quit, even if it's something you found valuable when you stopped a while back. This isn't the time to offer advice. It won't be taken very well.

But there's a lot you can do to ensure success. Giving up smoking is a major decision and a difficult task. Congratulate the person for taking that first step. Offer to help in any way you can, even if that means staying out of sight as much as possible! My wife says to this day that she would never have been able to quit if I hadn't taken the kids away for a week's fishing. She just wanted to be left alone.

The quitter **IS** going to be grumpy, grouchy, irritable, nasty, insulting and just plain miserable to be around. That goes with the territory for everyone but a saint, and there aren't too many of those around! Accept the trade-off of future good health and an environment free of smoke, ashtrays and stink. Assuming that he or she was lovable before trying to stop, he or she will be so again in just two or three weeks.

Giving up smoking is taking a big step towards improved health, including control of blood pressure and reduced risk of heart attack and stroke. Without going over the top about it, give the person frequent congratulations. Take note of the first cigarette-free week and subsequent landmarks.

Help to keep the quitter's mind off smoking. Suggest a film. Or a game of cards. Or a walk in the woods or along the beach.

Remember that it's just a matter of time, and try to help that time pass a bit faster during the cessation process. That person is worth it.

Giving up cigarettes was one of the most difficult things I have done in my life. It also helped save my life. I wish for you the same success.

More information

There's a lot of useful information for those who want to stop smoking cigarettes available on the internet from organisations around the world. Don't limit yourself to just one country!

American Cancer Society
www.cancer.org

American Heart Association and American Stroke Association
www.amhrt.org
www.strokeassociation.org

American Lung Association
www.lungusa.org

Action on Smoking and Health (ASH)
www.ash.org.uk

Centers for Disease Control and Prevention
Office on Smoking and Health
www.cdc.gov/tobacco

National Cancer Institute
www.cancer.gov

NHS Smoking Helpline
www.givingupsmoking.co.uk.

Nicotine Anonymous
www.nicotine-anonymous.org

Smokefree.gov (including information on state Quitlines)
www.smokefree.gov

Smoking Cessation Leadership Center
http://smokingcessationleadership.ucsf.edu/

Heart Foundation of Australia
www.heartfoundation.com.au

Chapter 9
The Electrolyte Balancing Act

We've all heard the same advice: cut back on salt and sodium in the diet. That advice has been around for so long, in fact, that most people just accept it at face value, assuming that taking the saltcellar off the dinner table will cause blood pressure to come down and hearts to get healthier. Well, it's just not that simple. We have to take sodium restriction recommendations with the proverbial pinch of salt.

Without going into a lot of scientific details that you really don't need to know, suffice to say that sodium is one of four electrolytes, along with calcium, magnesium and potassium, needed by the body to achieve its daily functions. Every time the heart beats or muscles contract, electrolytes come into play. Without the proper combination, the heart would stop beating and muscles would either go rigid or flaccid. Messages pass through our nervous system as sodium enters a nerve cell and potassium exits. After the message is transmitted, sodium leaves the cell. Without that so-called 'sodium-potassium pump' our bodies would pretty much shut down. Similarly, we can't do without calcium and magnesium either.

Salt makes our foods taste better. And most of us living in the West consume too much of it. No question about that. We'd get all the sodium we need from just one teaspoon of salt or sodium chloride. But we like to put it into the water before boiling potatoes or making pasta, and we sprinkle on more when we sit down to eat. And 75 per cent of all the sodium in the diet comes from processed foods that contain not only sodium chloride but also a whole family of sodium compounds to make those foods taste good and to make them last longer on the supermarket shelves and in our larders, breadbins and refrigerators.

The other electrolytes, unfortunately, don't taste as good. We don't sprinkle potassium chloride on our popcorn or put it on the rims of margarita glasses, though as we'll see we might want to get into the habit of consuming more potassium as well as more calcium and magnesium.

Should everyone restrict salt and sodium?

Heart authorities in the US, UK, Australia and just about everywhere else urge citizens to cut back, right back, on their salt and sodium consumption. For many people, that can help control hypertension. That's especially true for black people and older men and women, all of whom are more salt sensitive than others. About 25 to 50 per cent, perhaps more, of those with hypertension – not necessarily mildly raised blood pressure – are sodium sensitive. Black people have a higher rate of sodium sensitivity. But that leaves a lot of men and women who are not sensitive to sodium.

There's no doubt that genetics plays a major role in how the body deals with sodium. The way our kidneys handle salt and sodium makes the difference. Let's look at a laboratory experiment carried out on rats that were bred to be either sodium sensitive or sodium-resistant. The blood pressure of sensitive rats rose quickly when fed a diet high in sodium. But that of sodium-resistant rats was not affected. When the kidney of a rat that has normal blood pressure when fed salt was transplanted into a sodium-sensitive rat, the recipient rat's BP went up. Conversely, when a sodium-sensitive rat got a kidney from a rodent that was sodium resistant, BP went down.

In a nutshell, salt and other sodium compounds are involved in a chemical sequence initiated in the kidneys that ends with the production of a substance, angiotensin, that raises blood pressure. In fact, some of the blood pressure drugs that doctors prescribe block the action of angiotensin. The more sensitive one is to sodium, the more angiotensin is made in the kidney, the more sodium is stored in the body, and the more water is retained in the body's tissues. All this raises blood pressure.

The anti-salt zealots like to point to the famous International Intersalt Study, the most comprehensive effort undertaken thus far. Researchers looked at blood pressure and sodium intake in 32 countries. For the most part, the results revealed little link between sodium intake and hypertension in people around the world. That said, however, people in countries that had extremely high salt intake tended to have higher blood pressure, while those with very little salt in their diets had lower levels. But those are the extremes. For most people in most countries, there was little association between salt/sodium consumption and blood pressure. And people in Thailand who traditionally eat very salty diets had relatively low BP.

Here's the basic truth. Take a person with normal blood pressure, feed him or her excessive amounts of salt and blood pressure will go up. Bring that salt intake back down and BP goes down along with it. That physiological fact was even demonstrated in chimpanzees, animals pretty similar to us in many ways. But, again, we're talking about extremes. These and other findings suggest that unless sodium is very severely limited, most people will not see any improvement. Any drop in blood pressure, on average, will be clinically insignificant. Just for the fun of it, let's look a little closer at that chimp study, carried out by Australian scientists in Gabon, Africa.

Chimpanzees naturally consume a diet consisting mostly of fruit and vegetable matter. Half the chimps in the study were given a liquid that provided up to 15g of salt daily, a massive amount. After 20 months on the salt-laced diet, seven of the thirteen chimps showed a big increase in both systolic and diastolic BP. But three chimps showed no change at all and three didn't drink all the salt solution. Still, the conclusion was that salt raises BP.

Bear in mind that data in all such studies reflect averages. Even in a population where salt intake is very high, only certain individuals will show a rise in blood pressure. The majority will have a normal blood pressure, even if they consume the same amount of salt. But when the people who play with statistics take those data and crunch them all together, they can find *on average* that reduced salt/sodium intake lowers BP. Statistics may show, to exaggerate my point just a bit, that the average family has 2.2 children, but I've yet to see a cot or pushchair containing 0.2 of a child! Forget those averages, let's talk instead about real, individual men and women.

Let's look at just one of the many studies carried on with real, human subjects. For three years, 841 men and women were observed for the blood-pressure-lowering effects of diet. Some restricted sodium, some cut back on calories and others reduced both sodium and calories. The group that saw the biggest drop in blood pressure was that one that reduced its calorie intake. Those cutting back on sodium alone showed very little difference.

Within those groups, however, were men and women who were very sensitive to sodium. Salt/sodium sensitivity is a very real thing. In fact, researchers are now trying to develop a test for such sensitivity so that doctors know which patients need sodium restriction and which do not, rather than prescribing it for everyone. That test is still in the future. But the zealots say we don't need such a test because if everyone greatly restricted sodium intake, some would profit and society would be the better for it. Maybe some day we'll have that sensitivity test, and maybe not. In the meantime, we do know that black people, older individuals, those who are overweight, and those consuming little dietary fibre are more likely to be sensitive.

The *British Medical Journal* in 2002 published a review of 11 trials of interventions aimed at reducing dietary salt intake. Tens of thousands of subjects were involved, with and without hypertension. Follow-up ranged from six months to seven years, comparing the reduction in blood pressure of those advised to restrict salt intake with control groups – people not given that advice. The average difference was a mere 1.1mgHg systolic BP and 0.6mgHg diastolic BP.

In a commentary in the publication *Journal Watch*, the reviewing physician, Dr Keith Marton, wrote that, 'These interventions were highly restrictive and, as such, unlikely to be useful in primary care. Thus, the mild effect of dietary salt restriction on BP hardly seems worth the effort, especially given the apparent lack of significant effect on overall health.'

But Dr Marton also noted that 'these results do not rule out the possibility that an individual patient occasionally will have a more substantial response to salt restriction'. Such individuals are most likely to be black, overweight, older and hypertensive, since those men and women are more often salt sensitive. And data reported in 2005 from the University of Miami, in Florida, indicate that women may become more salt sensitive as they enter their postmenopausal years.

How can you tell if restricting your sodium intake would lower your BP? Experiment. Try testing yourself. Measure your blood pressure for a few days in a row. Cut back on processed foods, don't add salt when cooking, and put the saltcellar away. Do that for a few weeks and retest your BP. See if you benefit. If so, terrific. If not, there are other ways of lowering BP.

It may even be possible that a low-salt diet can do more harm than good. Dr Brent Egan, then at the Medical College of Wisconsin, in Milwaukee, found that a low-salt diet will not reduce BP in 50 per cent of people with higher-than-normal pressures and in 80 per cent of those with more normal pressures. In fact, for some people, salt restriction may actually result in higher blood pressure!

Even more disturbing was a study linking low sodium consumption with an increase in heart attack risk. Working with hypertensive men at the Albert Einstein College of Medicine, in New York City, Dr Michael Alderman detected an unexpectedly high incidence of heart attacks in those with low amounts of salt in their urine, reflecting their dietary restrictions. The study followed nearly 2,000 men for almost four years. More than four times as many heart attacks occurred in men with the lowest amounts of sodium in their urine compared with men with the highest amounts of urinary sodium.

Dr Alderman also studied more than 1,000 hypertensive women, but only nine of them suffered heart attacks during the study period, too small a number to draw any conclusions. Among the men, there were 46 heart attacks.

These data don't mean that everyone should rush out and start gobbling salt. The patients involved had significant hypertension and other factors to consider. But the findings do cast a big shadow on blanket recommendations that everyone should severely restrict their sodium consumption.

So what are doctors and their patients to do? Dr Egan takes a very practical approach with his own patients. He has them monitor their blood pressures for a week before starting a low-salt diet in order to establish that baseline. Then they keep track of their blood pressure after cutting back on salt. If there is no reduction in blood pressure after one to two months, Dr Egan tells them to discontinue salt restriction. After all, why follow a prescription that doesn't work, any more than a doctor would have a patient continue to take a drug that didn't achieve the desired effect.

Taking a moderate stance

As the old saying goes, all things in moderation. And the same advice should be given regarding salt and sodium intake. Practically all of us in the US, UK and elsewhere eat way too much. Even if becoming more moderate doesn't lower BP, there are other benefits including an easing of burden on the kidneys and lessening water retention. The vast majority of weight loss when starting a diet comes from water loss. Cut back – reasonably – on salt and sodium-rich foods and that water and weight loss can be permanent. Moderation, not restriction.

My wife and I enjoyed a weekend getaway at a Japanese hotel in Los Angeles featuring an authentic Japanese lifestyle, including the room, the grounds, a plunge pool and hot baths, Shiatsu massage, and typical food for breakfast, lunch and dinner. Japanese foods are notorious for their high salt content. By the end of the weekend, we couldn't remove the rings from our water-swollen fingers. Wow, what a dramatic demonstration of excess consumption. It's no surprise that the Japanese suffer a high rate of hypertension and strokes.

So how can we cut back so that we can still enjoy our foods? First of all, understand that we have become used to a high-salt diet. After two to three weeks, the urge to salt everything on the plate passes, and after a couple of months one begins to enjoy the natural flavours of foods and finds that the kinds of foods previously consumed taste overly salty.

Even the water we drink contains some sodium, but only about one per cent of our total consumption. Obviously, we don't want to restrict our water drinking. Next, foods in their natural state, even fruits and vegetables and, more notably, dairy foods provide about 12 per cent of intake. Surely we don't want to eliminate any of those healthy foods. The saltcellar on the table adds 6 per cent and cooking contributes 5 per cent. So where does the majority of salt and sodium come from? A whopping 75–77 per cent is in processed, manufactured and pre-packed foods, and meals eaten in fast-food restaurants. That's where we need to cut back. But we want to do so selectively.

Bread is made with salt, even though it doesn't taste salty. Try eating low-salt or salt-free bread and you're in for a horrible experience. The stuff tastes like cardboard. No flavour whatsoever. Try to make those kinds of changes and you're doomed to failure.

Start, instead, with 'baby steps'. If a recipe calls for 800g of tinned tomatoes, use a 400g tin of ordinary tomatoes and another 400g tin of salt-free tomatoes. You eliminate half the salt and virtually none of the flavour. Use the same approach for most other tinned and processed foods. As time goes by, and your taste buds change, you'll be able to switch to more and more low-salt foods. It's pretty easy to see how much sodium is in a given processed food, since the quantity per serving is listed on the label.

Staying away from fast-food restaurants is healthy for many reasons beyond salt reductions. You'll also slash your consumption of total fat, saturated fat and trans fats, as well as calories. The US has made some very fine contributions to the world, but fast-food restaurants are not among them. I was saddened during a month-long trip to China in 2005 to see streets lined with McDonald's, Pizza Hut and KFC Fried Chicken restaurants. The Chinese love KFC the most, savouring deep-fried chicken skin. Sound disgusting? Remember that Peking duck feasts offer slices of the skin with very little meat; most of the carcass is discarded.

I realise that my next suggestion will sound virtually revolutionary – if not completely out of the realm of reason and all practicality. Try cooking and eating more at home, enjoying home-made foods. Again, start with 'baby steps' of perhaps one extra home-made meal per week. I think some of my recipe suggestions in Chapter 17 will make your mouth water and tempt you to try to prepare those dishes, many if not most of which are designed to lower blood pressure, not because of what they don't contain but what they do, in keeping with a Mediterranean diet. But more about that later.

Right now we're talking about sodium and, don't forget, those other electrolytes. It's difficult, I believe, to accurately keep track of the actual amount of salt/sodium we eat daily. I thing that merely following the suggestions above to whatever extent you are willing to go will be adequate for the average person, especially if extreme sodium restriction is not mandatory, as might be the case for someone with severe hypertension, the sort of patient who would often be prescribed a minimum of two and up to five different drugs to control their BP. For the record, the maximum daily amount of sodium recommended for the average UK adult is 2.4g (2.8g per day for men and 2g per day for women). That's 6g of salt daily, on average – about one teaspoonful. Other than perhaps some very diligent dietitians, I doubt that many individuals have any idea as to how much salt/sodium they consume daily or what it would mean to cut back to suggested levels. That's why I put forth my ideas on how to rather painlessly reduce intake in the paragraphs above. So what can we do beyond a reasonable, moderate sodium cutback?

Do you use a water softener? You might be getting a lot of sodium from the water you're drinking. That might be particularly important if you're sodium sensitive. Have an unsoftened water system for drinking and cooking purposes. Water softening systems that use potassium- rather than sodium-based softening agents might be a good idea, giving you an additional source of that mineral, another electrolyte in the balancing act, unless your doctor has advised you to limit potassium if you have problems with your kidney function.

Looking for electrolytes

It is my fervent belief that cutting back on salt and sodium offer just a small, though useful, start to improving our blood pressure status. Probably far more important is making a real effort to increase the other electrolytes: calcium, magnesium and potassium. In fact, I think that most of the benefit in switching from salt to a salt substitute at the dinner table or for food preparation comes not from cutting back on the sodium chloride but, rather, from increasing consumption of potassium chloride.

Potassium

In fact, most national health authorities now recommend increased potassium consumption along with advice to cut back on sodium. That's true for the UK Food Standards Agency, US Dietary Guidelines Advisory Committee, the National Academy of Sciences' Food and Nutrition Board, the National Heart, Lung and Blood Institute of the National Institutes of Health, the American Heart Association, Health Canada and the Australian Heart Foundation. The reason for such unanimity is simple: the science just can't be denied. Potassium is a chemical element that helps maintain the normal functioning of the heart and nervous system.

In 1991, University of Pennsylvania researchers found that just ten days of potassium restriction resulted in a rise in blood pressure, whether one had normal or raised BP to begin with. A 12-year study of Californian adults suggested that high potassium intake protects against stroke, the worst result of hypertension. For men in that study, those with low potassium intakes were at 2.6 times more risk of stroke than those who consumed a lot of potassium-rich foods. For women, low intake multiplied the risk nearly five times.

Potassium restriction was also associated with sodium retention and with calcium depletion in various studies. In fact, the converse is true, giving a good explanation as to why potassium works so well. The mineral causes the body to excrete more sodium in the urine, the same mode of action achieved with anti-hypertensive drugs called thiazide diuretics (see page 249). Potassium also seems to correct salt sensitivity.

Doctors at the famed Johns Hopkins Medical Center, in Baltimore, Maryland, investigated the potential of adding potassium to the diet in 1994. They gave potassium supplements to one group of African-Americans, known to have a high incidence of salt sensitivity and hypertension, and a placebo to a similar group. Both groups had what would be termed high-normal blood pressure or pre-hypertension (see page 2) – 125/77 in one group and 127/78 in the other.

At the end of three weeks – just three weeks! – systolic BP dropped an average of 6.9 points in those taking the potassium supplements, and diastolic readings tumbled by 2.5 points. That's a lot of improvement for little effort.

More recently, British researchers gave half of a group of 69 healthy volunteers potassium supplements three times daily, providing the amount of the mineral found in five servings of fruits and vegetables. The others got a placebo. At the end of the six-week trial, those getting the potassium enjoyed a decline in systolic BP of 7.60mgHg and a drop of 6.46mgHg in diastolic BP. Improvement occurred gradually over the six-week period.

Again, there's no doubt in the scientific and medical communities that potassium is one answer to the blood pressure problems in Western countries around the world.

And there are additional benefits from making sure one's diet is rich in potassium. The mineral helps prevent kidney stones and heartbeat disturbances called arrhythmias. It also keeps the bones strong by neutralising acids in the bloodstream that leach calcium from bone.

Palaeontologists studying the eating habits of our early ancestors have universally found that their diet was low in sodium and high in potassium. They ate a lot of very lean meat whenever they could get it and relied heavily on fruits and vegetables. Conversely, our modern diet is high in sodium and low in potassium, since we consume sodium-rich processed foods and little in the way of those fruits and veggies.

Sadly, other than vegetarians – who still might consume too much sodium, by the way – most of us consume too little potassium because we just don't eat enough fruits and vegetables. That's been shown to be the case in the UK, US, Canada, Australia and Europe. Typically, the most frequently consumed vegetable is the potato – as chips or crisps.

So how much potassium should we aim for? Recommendations call for at least 4.7g daily to lower blood pressure, blunt the effects of salt, reduce the risk of kidney stones and bone loss, and stabilise heartbeat. Round that off to 5g. And many, if not most, authorities would agree that you just can't consume too much of this 'miracle' mineral, although that doesn't mean going overboard with potassium supplements and potassium-containing salt substitutes. The only exceptions would be individuals with impaired kidney function or severe congestive heart failure. They should speak to their doctors before increasing potassium intake.

And it's really easy to do just by paying a little more attention to the diet. Because the health benefits of potassium are getting more attention, many food companies are listing the amount of the mineral on food labels when that food offers a significant contribution. Raw foods don't necessarily carry nutrition information labels. So opposite is a chart of some of the best sources of potassium.

Surely, in that list, there must be some foods that start your mouth watering! Why not add some of them to your shopping list right now. And be sure to include some dried fruits such as apricots and raisins that you can keep in your car, handbag

FOOD	AMOUNT	POTASSIUM (mg)
Sweet potato/yam	150g	950
Honeydew melon	½ melon	940
Squash	150g	900
Potato (baked)	1 medium	844
Avocado	½ medium	680
Dried figs	5 whole	666
Prunes	10 medium	626
Dates	10 whole	541
Tomato pureé	100ml	525
Dried apricots	10 halves	482
Banana	1 medium	451
Cantaloupe	150g	450
Orange juice	100ml	450
Raisins	75g	375
Mango	1 medium	323
Orange	1 medium	250
Strawberries	150g	247

Meat

FOOD	AMOUNT	POTASSIUM (mg)
Grilled lean beef	100g	426
Lamb sirloin	100g	186
Grilled pork loin	100g	375

Seasonings

FOOD	AMOUNT	POTASSIUM (mg)
Cream of tartar	1 teaspoon	495

Salt substitutes

FOOD	AMOUNT	POTASSIUM (mg)
Low-sodium salt	1 teaspoon	1,500
Salt substitute	1 teaspoon	2,800

or office for handy, healthy snacks. Aim for a potassium intake of at least 3,500mg daily, ideally 4,700mg (4.7g).

Notice that those salt substitutes provide a whopping amount of potassium, using potassium chloride instead of sodium chloride. Just replacing the saltcellar with one of those substitutes, or using both intermittently, will help boost your potassium intake and lower your blood pressure. Don't like the taste? Add some to foods as they're cooking and you won't even notice. Then use just a tiny sprinkle of regular table salt when eating.

Forget the potassium supplement tablets available in many stores and pharmacies. One potassium gluconate tablet is listed on a bottle I checked as 550mg. But read the information on the back and you'll learn, as I did, that the tablet actually contains only 90mg of actual potassium. You can get five times as much as that from a glass of orange juice.

Calcium

Dr David McCarron of the Oregon Health Sciences University, in Portland, pioneered the research showing that insufficient calcium in the diet could be as important, or even more so, as consuming too much sodium. And additional studies have corroborated his initial findings.

In a project at Johns Hopkins Medical Center, in Baltimore, Maryland, researchers found that 23 women who took 1.5g or 2g of calcium carbonate supplements daily throughout pregnancy decreased diastolic blood pressure by 4–7mmHg. The higher calcium dose yielded the more dramatic BP improvements. Results were the same in both white and black women.

The research has been international. Dutch investigators reported lowering blood pressure with calcium supplements. One gram daily reduced diastolic BP by 3.1mmHg in just six weeks. In one of the largest studies of its kind, California medical scientists found that every gram of calcium consumed per day lowered the risk of high blood pressure by 12 per cent on average for the 6,634 men and women participating. Benefits are greater for certain individuals. Those under 40 have 25 per cent less risk per gram of calcium. Lean men and women demonstrate an 18 per cent risk reduction. Those drinking less than one alcoholic beverage per day get a 16 per cent cut in hypertension risk per calcium gram consumed.

How does calcium work its wonders on blood pressure? This gets a bit technical. The mineral reduces the concentration of parathyroid hormone in the blood; that hormone regulates calcium metabolism. In turn, that might lower calcium concentrations in the body's cells and slow calcium from entering arteries. Calcium in the arteries affects the tone of the vessel, thus potentially leading to higher blood pressure as the artery stiffens.

The calcium supplements a woman takes during pregnancy may leave a lasting benefit by lowering her child's blood pressure. Toddlers whose mothers took pre-natal calcium supplements had lower BPs than those whose mothers did not. According to the lead investigator of that study in Oregon, such calcium intake may help 'programme' fetal blood pressure, possibly with effects that last into adulthood.

View supplements as just that: an adjunct, not a replacement for dietary calcium. Fat-free and low-fat dairy foods, with the exception of cottage cheese, are excellent sources of calcium and belong in everyone's diet throughout life. Aim for two or even three servings a day. Don't like milk? Enjoy some yogurt. Or cheese. Even ice cream. Just be sure to choose the fat-free and/or low-fat varieties. Read the nutrition information labels on dairy foods and you'll see how easy it is to boost your intake of that mineral.

Some dietitians recommend tinned salmon as a calcium source. But that assumes that you'll mix the bones in with the fish as you make, say, a salmon salad sandwich. However, most people toss those bones away. And as for another frequent recommendation to eat a lot of green, leafy vegetables for their calcium content, bear two things in mind. First, few of us are likely to consume enough of those greens each and every day. Second, the calcium in greens is not as well absorbed as that in dairy foods.

All that said, the fact remains that the vast majority of adults will have to use supplements to get the 1,200–1,600mg women require both for bone health and blood pressure control and the 800mg men need. And there's another benefit shown for taking calcium supplements: they appear to lessen the risk of colorectal cancer by limiting rapid cellular growth in that area of the digestive tract.

What sort of calcium supplements should you choose? For bone health, find one that includes vitamin D, needed to build bone tissue. Many antacid products are made with calcium carbonate and add to the day's calcium intake.

Calcium carbonate is the least expensive source of calcium in supplements. Regardless of the form – carbonate, citrate or gluconate – read the label to determine how much of the actual mineral each tablet provides. Happily, some manufacturers are now offering calcium/magnesium supplements, which I highly recommend.

Magnesium

This mineral is the fourth electrolyte needed by the body. And, as with the other electrolytes other than sodium, we consume less than we should. Most nutritionists do not consider magnesium deficiency to be a major problem, since it's widely available in the food supply and many men and women get an additional amount by way of a multivitamin/mineral supplement. But that doesn't mean we get enough.

Magnesium aids in energy metabolism, promotes proper nerve function, and is involved with muscle activity. It also activates certain enzymes, stabilises cell structures, and is used for the body to make cell protein, fats and carbohydrates. Magnesium supplements are often recommended for muscle cramp and other ailments. But our main interest right now is in how this electrolyte can affect blood pressure.

Again, there's a lot of science to back up the notion that we all need to increase our magnesium intake. There have been quite a number of observations that certain world populations with higher magnesium consumption in their diet have reduced risk of hypertension. But until fairly recently there haven't been the kind of clinical studies that medical authorities need to make specific recommendations. Here are just three representative studies of just that kind of scientific investigation.

At Johns Hopkins Medical Center, in Baltimore, Maryland, doctors collected data from 20 trials that looked at the effects of magnesium supplementation on blood pressure. They pooled the data to form one 'megastudy' in what is termed a meta-analysis. In six of the studies, subjects had normal blood pressures; in the others, patients were hypertensive. The data came from 1,220 men and women, and the daily dose of magnesium ranged from 180 to 720mg.

Their conclusions are encouraging. For each 180mg increase in daily magnesium intake, systolic and diastolic blood pressure decreased by 4.3 and 2.3mmHg, respectively. Reductions in blood pressure were 'dose dependent'. That is to say, the more magnesium consumed, the greater the BP decline.

What about the impact of magnesium on the development of heart disease risk? Doctors at the University of Virginia Health System looked at the daily dietary magnesium intake in 7,172 men whose consumption ranged from 50.3 to 1138mg with an average of 268mg. During 30 years of follow-up, there were 1,431 cases of coronary heart disease (CHD), and within 15 years of dietary assessment the age-adjusted incidence of CHD fell significantly in those with the highest daily magnesium intake (340mg or more) compared to the lowest (186mg or less).

In a third study, published in 2004, low levels of magnesium in the blood were associated with an increased risk of stroke. Those low magnesium levels apparently trigger constriction of arteries and increase injury to the endothelium, the lining of arteries, which promotes the development and progression of heart disease. Those with the highest blood concentrations of magnesium had one-third the risk of those with the lowest levels.

US nutrition authorities recommend 420mg for adult men and 320mg for women as a minimum. Obviously, as we can see in the above studies, more is better. Aiming for 700mg is not beyond reason.

A major study monitored 4,637 men and women aged 18–30 for 15 years. Those in the top quarter in terms of magnesium consumption from foods and supplements were less likely to develop high blood pressure as well as other components of the metabolic syndrome that includes high triglycerides and insulin resistance, a precursor to diabetes.

Where do we get magnesium in the diet? A bit more than 20 per cent comes from dairy foods and another 15 per cent from meat. That's interesting, since those foods aren't particularly rich in magnesium, but we eat a lot of them in the West. Better choices for those desiring to boost their magnesium intakes would be a variety of plant foods such as beans, bananas, almonds, cashews and greens. Clams, by the way, are packed with magnesium; five small ones provide a whopping 112mg.

I think everyone looking to keep blood pressure down should seriously consider magnesium supplements. Daily supplementation of at least 300mg seems reasonable. That's what I personally take. My supplement contains 300mg of calcium and 150mg of magnesium per tablet, and I take two daily.

The electrolyte balance

In summary, salt/sodium restriction is difficult to achieve and, when viewed alone, not terribly effective in lowering blood pressure. Few individuals are willing to eat a very bland ultra-low-salt diet for the rest of their lives. And small cutbacks, while advisable, won't do much good if that's all one does.

The answer, I believe, and many agree, is to seek an electrolyte balance of sodium, potassium, calcium and magnesium. This appears to be the winning formula for blood pressure control.

Chapter 10

To Drink or Not to Drink?

In the past, doctors automatically instructed patients with high blood pressure to stop drinking alcohol. I clearly remember when my own cardiologist, who had hypertension, was told by his cardiologist, 'No more booze.' I also remember thinking that I'd have a tougher time giving up my cocktail before dinner or wine with the meal than cutting right back on fat, as I was doing to control my high cholesterol.

Happily, today doctors around the world recognise the potential benefits of alcohol consumption, even for those with blood pressure problems. In fact, moderate drinking may actually be good for them. The watchword, of course, is moderation, as it should be for everyone.

More than a French paradox

The benefits of alcohol consumption first got public attention when it was noted that the French, who had a very low incidence of heart disease, regularly consumed wine, particularly red wine, with their meals. In fact, the French drink a lot of wine, more than they should, and it wasn't noted that France has one of the world's highest incidence rates of cirrhosis of the liver.

Since the time of those first reports, researchers around the world have contributed to the now massive body of knowledge regarding the health benefits of alcohol. Looking at mortality rates, it became obvious early on that those who enjoyed a drink or two daily had a lower incidence of cardiovascular disease and lived longer than those who did not drink.

Critics of that observation suggested that investigations included those who had quit drinking owing to illnesses, and that those illnesses, in fact, were responsible for earlier deaths. But when research efforts were refined to exclude such men and women, and focused only on those who had never consumed alcohol, the protective effect of alcohol held up.

Then it became a question, almost a noisy argument, about what kind of alcohol was best.

Was it the red wine favoured by the French? Wine merchants touted that, of course. Or was it the beer enjoyed by Germans and others? And what about the spirits preferred by those sipping a martini?

First, let's dispel the superiority of wine in general and red wine in particular. According to Greek researchers in 2005, drinking red wine reduced arterial stiffness in the heart disease patients in their study. As Dr Emmanouil Karatzis of Athens said, 'This is very important considering the fact that patients' vessels are already stiff and this is a major cause of increased blood pressure and consequently increased risk for cardiovascular events.' But those benefits were also enjoyed by those who drank alcohol-free red wine.

This added one more bit of data to the argument that, in fact, the benefits of red wine come from the type of chemicals called polyphenols and flavonoids, found in the skins of red grapes. Those chemicals are not found in white wine, since grape skins are removed at the start of the fermentation process. But one can very easily get those polyphenols and flavonoids from red grape juice or pomegranate juice. Or, for that matter, from green tea and a wide variety of fruits and vegetables. Or beer.

My wife, in fact, enjoys a Cosmopolitan cocktail now and then, and I make it for her with a splash of pomegranate juice.

And that brings me back to the issue of what alcoholic beverage is best for heart protection. The short, simple answer is that all kinds of alcoholic drinks provide benefits. It turns out that alcohol itself yields good things for the body.

More about that in a moment. But first, what about all those studies showing that men and women who drink wine regularly, rather than either beer or spirits, have a significantly lower rate of heart disease and suffer fewer heart attacks and strokes? It turns out that it's more about the lifestyles of wine lovers rather than the wine itself.

There have actually been quite a few papers in the medical literature that make that point. One of the most recent came from Danish investigators in 2006. Wine drinkers in the Copenhagen study have healthier diets than people who prefer beer. They buy and eat more fruits, vegetables, olives, low-fat cheese and cooking oil. Beer drinkers there, on the other hand, consume fast food, soft drinks, sugar and saturated and trans fats. To add insult to injury, those wine drinkers were better educated, healthier and leaner. Californian investigators have come to the same conclusion about wine drinkers in that state. And, it appears, the same applies to French wine drinkers.

The benefits of alcohol

Alcohol, whatever your drink preference, works its wonders in many ways. The most notable is raising levels of the protective 'good' HDL cholesterol. This is pretty much a linear phenomenon. Up to a certain point, the more one drinks, the higher the HDL goes. But, of course, there's the standing caveat of moderation, which I'll define shortly.

Recent investigations have also revealed that alcohol reduces inflammation in the arteries. Doctors have noted that those with heart disease have higher levels of inflammation and, conversely, those with little inflammation are at lessened risk of developing the disease and/or suffering a heart attack or stroke.

In fact, there are more than 1,000 English language papers analysing the relationship between alcohol usage and the incidence of stroke. Light to moderate alcohol intake has been reported to reduce the rate of all types of stroke, based on a long-term, on-going study of doctors conducted at Harvard University. Grouped together, studies carried out between 1966 and 2002 on the link between alcohol and stroke show a decreased risk. And such findings have been reported around the world. One of the most recent comes from Columbia University, in New York. There doctors worked with 3,176 mostly Hispanic subjects who were divided up into men and women who reported:

- drinking no alcohol during the previous year,
- moderate consumption of at least one alcoholic drink per month but no more than two alcoholic drinks a day,
- intermediate intake of more than two but fewer than five alcoholic drinks a day or
- heavy intake of at least five alcoholic drinks a day.

During the years of follow-up, moderate drinkers showed a 33 per cent lower risk of stroke compared with those who had consumed no alcohol during the previous year.

Alcohol also improves insulin resistance, a component of so-called metabolic syndrome, which predisposes men and women to diabetes and increased risk of heart attack and stroke (see page 55). It improves the ability of arteries to dilate to allow for greater blood flow when needed. And alcohol reduces risk of developing blood clots by way of cutting down levels of fibrinogen, a component in the clotting process.

But what about hypertensive patients specifically? While most studies in the medical literature have involved patients with various levels of blood pressure rather than focusing on hypertensive individuals, it appears alcohol's benefits extend to the latter as well. A 2004 study, for example, showed that light to moderate alcohol intake appears to be associated with reduced cardiovascular disease mortality, from both heart attack and stroke. That research was also conducted with doctors in the Harvard University study.

How much? How often?

A lot of people use the word 'moderate' without giving much thought to a precise meaning or definition. When it comes to alcohol consumption, medical authorities are virtually un-animous in their recommendations. Moderate means no more than one drink daily for women and two drinks a day for men. One drink is defined as half a pint of beer (less for brews higher than usual alcohol content), one glass of wine containing 12 per cent alcohol by volume (12%ABV) or a standard 25ml measure of spirits ranging from 35 to 40%ABV, such as whisky, gin, vodka or bourbon.

Consumption frequency also comes into play. Based on a giant collection of data from 32,826 women and 18,225 men, Harvard researchers concluded that drinking at least three to four days a week is associated with lowered risk of heart attack. The lowest risk was seen in those drinking three to seven days a week. Another investigation revealed drinking three to six alcoholic beverages weekly lowers the tendency of blood to clot, but that there was no additional benefit beyond six weekly drinks.

Truth be told, however, heavier alcohol consumption provides other protective benefits against heart disease. Almost grudgingly, a commentary in the British medical journal *The Lancet* in 2005 pointed out that during autopsies, the coronary arteries of alcoholics are frequently relatively 'clean', indicating a linear level of protection, whether from high HDL cholesterol, reduced levels of inflammation or whatever.

But the authors of that commentary, from the University of Auckland, in New Zealand, also note the significant negative effects of heavy alcohol usage. Once again, medical authorities are unanimous in strongly warning against heavy drinking.

In studies corroborated again and again all over the globe, as men and women go from being non-drinkers, to light to moderate drinkers, their risk of cardiovascular disease decreases. But as study populations in general, and individuals in particular, graduate from moderate to heavy drinking risk of all-cause mortality goes up. Canadian research has shown that women, in particular, appear to be more at risk of hypertension when alcohol consumption goes beyond moderate levels. In that 2006 investigation, doctors found that heavy alcohol use raised blood pressure levels throughout both day and night.

And the heavier the drinking the greater the risk. Heavy drinkers are at increased risk of alcoholism as well as accidental injuries and deaths, especially on the roads. Cirrhosis of the liver becomes more likely, too. And heart muscle, which is protected by light to moderate drinking, is damaged by heavy alcohol intake. Binge drinking, defined as five or more units in a single day, poses particular ill effects.

Alcohol and blood pressure

A report issued by the American Heart Association in 2006 points to clinical trials showing that reducing excess alcohol consumption lowers both systolic and diastolic blood pressure. However, the AHA says, evidence supports the fact that moderate alcohol intake is effective in lowering blood pressure. The group concludes that alcohol consumption should be limited to no more than two drinks a day for men and one drink for women.

The Australian Heart Foundation in 2004 stated that 'those drinking the equivalent of three or more glasses of beer a day have three times the prevalence of hypertension compared to patients who abstain'. The AHF refers to studies showing evidence that alcohol can raise blood pressure and interfere with the action of hypertensive drugs. Heavier drinking, the group says, increases the risk of stroke, heart failure and arrhythmias (disturbances in heartbeat). Their recommendation: 'Patients with hypertension who drink alcohol should be advised to avoid binge drinking and limit their usual alcohol intake to one (if female) or two (if male) standard drinks per day.'

There has been considerable discussion in the world's medical literature and at medical conferences as to whether doctors should actually advocate initiation of alcohol consumption for those patients who do not currently drink. Certainly there is unequivocal proof of the cardiovascular benefits. But there is also unequivocal proof of the potential downside of drinking, both for the individual and for society as a whole. The horrors of deaths both to drinking drivers and their victims come vividly and dramatically to mind, as does the sociological impact of alcoholism on the individual and his or her family.

Doctors conclude, and I strongly agree, that if you currently enjoy light to moderate alcohol consumption, continue to do so. But if you are a non-drinker, do not begin to drink just to protect your heart. Whether you lift a glass of an alcoholic or non-alcoholic beverage, I end this chapter with a toast.

To good health and happiness!

Chapter 11

The Cholesterol/ Blood Pressure Connection

What is a chapter on cholesterol doing in a book on blood pressure? For openers, raised cholesterol levels in the blood represent one of the 'Big Three' risk factors for cardiovascular disease, along with blood pressure and cigarette smoking. But there's another reason. It now appears that blood pressure and cholesterol are more closely related than anyone previously thought.

In 2005, research demonstrated that lowering blood pressure brings cholesterol counts down at the same time. The following year, doctors examining data from an on-going study of thousands of women found that high cholesterol tests predict future hypertension. The higher a woman's cholesterol during middle age, the more likely she'll later develop high blood pressure. Women in this particular subset of the investigation were at least 45 years old in 1992, and none had high cholesterol or raised blood pressure. After nearly 11 years, 4,593 women – nearly one-third – had developed high blood pressure. Those with the highest ratio of total cholesterol to protective 'good' HDL cholesterol had a 34 per cent greater risk of hypertension. Conversely, women with high HDL counts had a 16 per cent lower than average risk. And, also in 2006, that link was extended to men by way of the Physicians' Health Study, a similar on-going investigation of thousands of men whose diets, lifestyle habits, and development and progression of disease is carefully monitored.

In this particular case, the study period was just over 14 years. During that time, 1,019 male doctors in a group of 3,110 developed hypertension. Harvard researchers then compared the cholesterol levels of those men with others whose blood pressure remained in the normal range. Men having the highest levels of total cholesterol were 23 per cent more likely to develop hypertension than men with the lowest counts. And men with the highest ratio of total cholesterol to HDL cholesterol had a 54 per cent greater risk of developing high blood pressure.

The message is simple. Whether you're a man or a woman, you kill two birds with one stone by getting your cholesterol under control. Reduce the risk posed by that factor and you cut the risk of developing hypertension later in life.

Having personally fought high cholesterol levels since 1984 at the time of my second coronary bypass surgery and written extensively on cholesterol itself, I think I'm in a good position to give you some sound advice. Back in 1984, my total cholesterol was dangerously high. By following the programme I developed it dropped to safe levels in just eight weeks. I shared my regimen with the world in 1987 with the book *The 8-Week Cholesterol Cure* and in the 2002 complete rewrite and update, *The New 8-Week Cholesterol Cure*.

Obviously, I can't cover all the details I discuss in those books, but I think I can give you enough information, at least to start with, to get you solidly on the road to cholesterol control in this chapter. The bottom line promise, as has been true since 1987, is that you can get your cholesterol down to safe levels in just eight weeks. The programme I'm going to outline has worked for millions of men and women and can work for you.

What is cholesterol?

That's still the first question most people ask. Simply stated, cholesterol is a chemical substance essential for bodily functions including digestion, manufacture of hormones, formation of cell walls and protection of nerve endings. We can't live without it. It's in practically every tissue of our bodies.

That's the good news. The bad news is that when there's too much cholesterol, it tends to cause a blockage in our arteries, leading to heart disease, heart attacks, and stroke. Cholesterol has also been linked with Alzheimer's disease.

The substance itself isn't soluble in water or, on a more practical level, in the bloodstream. So cholesterol is transported through the body in a variety of envelopes made of fat and protein, called lipoproteins. Cholesterol transported in a low-density lipoprotein envelope tends to be deposited in damaged regions of our arteries. That's a bad thing, so we call LDL (low-density lipoprotein) cholesterol 'bad'. But in the body's system of balances, we also have cholesterol transported out of those arteries and removed from the bloodstream by HDL (high-density lipoprotein). We call HDL 'good' cholesterol.

Most of the cholesterol in our bloodstream, about 80 per cent of it, is made by the body itself, principally in the liver. In an ideal situation, there would be a proper balance of the LDL and HDL cholesterol, not too much of the LDL and enough HDL. But nearly 50 per cent of men and women inherit a family gene that results in the production of too much LDL and too little HDL. Even with a heart-healthy lifestyle of diet and exercise, such people will still have a cholesterol level that predisposes them to develop cardiovascular disease and eventually heart attacks and strokes.

The other fatty substances floating around in our blood are the triglycerides. These fats are used by the body for energy and come from the foods we eat. Here, too, some of us just naturally have too much, and our lifestyles boost levels even more, resulting in a risk factor independent from cholesterol.

Wouldn't it be terrific if we could simply 'tell' our livers not to make so much of the bad LDL cholesterol and make more of the good HDL cholesterol instead? And it would be even better if we could cut down the amount of triglycerides in our blood as well. The good news is that we can do just that, without having to resort to prescription drugs.

First things first: get tested

You have no idea whether you have a high cholesterol level or not without testing for it in the blood. Perversely, high cholesterol causes no symptoms and someone who is obese and sedentary may have a relatively low level while a lean, athletic person's cholesterol might be dangerously high. Not fair, is it?

Fortunately, cholesterol testing is quite simple and provides vital information for us to fight against heart disease. Simply schedule a day and time to visit your GP's surgery or health clinic, preferably in the morning before you've eaten anything that day. You'll want to get what doctors called a 'lipid panel', which consists of measurement of total cholesterol (TC), LDL cholesterol, HDL cholesterol, the ratio of total to good cholesterol and triglycerides (TG). Request a measurement of your glucose levels as well; they should be less than 6, and ideally just under 5. You can get those tests done at the same time you have your blood fats measured. You should have the results in just a few days.

Medical authorities state that TC should ideally be no more than 5.2mmol/l. That's fine, I suppose, if there's no family history of heart disease and if you have no other risk factors going on at the same time, such as raised blood pressure, sedentary lifestyle, smoking, diabetes and being overweight. If you have heart disease or diabetes, for example, you should aim for 5mmol/l maximum. The lower you can get your TC, the better. Risk begins to increase well before the cut-offs above.

Levels of LDL should be less than 3.5mmol/l. Again, the lower the better. If you have heart disease or diabetes you should aim for 3mmol/l. Conversely, we want HDL to be as high as possible, with women's levels no lower than 1.1mmol/l and men's no lower than 1.2mmol/l. The ratio of TC/HDL has been shown to be an even more accurate predictor of risk than TC or LDL alone. We want your ratio to be no more than 4.5 for men and 4.0 for women. Finally, TG counts should be under 2mmol/l, and ideally down to about 1.1 or so.

I strongly suggest that you ask your doctor to send a printed copy of your report so you can keep it in a file and use it for comparison in the years to come. Don't accept a statement that 'everything's okay'. Learn what your actual numbers are. Each of us should maintain a personal health file in our homes. Put your cholesterol report in that file, along with your blood pressure measurement and other medical information. (When did you last have a booster injection for tetanus, for example?)

Okay, you've had your test and you see that your numbers need improvement. No problem. Controlling cholesterol levels – all your lipids – is far easier today than it was back in 1984 when I began my own efforts. Let's start with a cholesterol-lowering diet.

Heart-healthy diet

Essentially, the ideal diet for controlling blood pressure, as described in Chapter 12, is just what you need for cholesterol lowering and maintenance as well. So here I'll just discuss a few of the principal points that particularly pertain to cholesterol.

It turns out that not all fats and oils are the villains the medical community thought them to be in the 1980s. Recommendations then were to reduce all fats. Today we've refined that, knowing that it's only the saturated and trans fats and oils we need to limit.

Saturated fats are found in meats and dairy foods and in palm kernel and coconut oils. But that doesn't mean we have to become vegetarians. Simply opt for lean cuts of beef, lamb and pork, and fat-free or at least low-fat dairy products. Read food labels to avoid palm kernel and coconut oils. Interestingly, while palm oil is as high in saturated fat as butter, the principal fatty acid doesn't affect cholesterol levels in our blood.

A very recent study in the *American Journal of Clinical Nutrition* showed that substituting some of the carbohydrates in the diet with lean red meat actually lowered blood pressure. Carbs replaced included white bread, pasta, white rice, and cakes and cookies. Ultimately it's a question of balance. But this study shows that there's no need to exclude lean cuts of red meat from a heart-smart diet.

The last thing you'd want to do is eliminate dairy foods in a misguided effort to avoid saturated fat or to lower calorie intake. We all need calcium for good bone health and for a variety of body functions. Moreover, it appears that those who consume the most low-fat dairy foods have half the incidence of hypertension, according to Spanish investigators who looked at the diets of nearly 6,000 well-educated men and women who had normal blood pressure at the beginning of the study and who developed hypertension over a 27-month study.

My first thought in reading the article was that it must be the calcium in dairy, but that, it turned out, was not the case at all, even though calcium itself is, indeed, part of the electrolyte balance needed to control blood pressure. In this study, however, those getting as much calcium from other sources did not enjoy the same protection. Nor did those who consumed whole-fat dairy foods. Only the low-fat dairy products provided blood pressure maintenance.

Trans fats are found in manufactured and processed foods such as cream crackers, biscuits and other bakery products, and in deep-fried fast foods. When shopping, look for 'partially hydrogenated' oils in the ingredients list. The process of hydrogenation, carried out to lengthen shelf life and improve taste, produces the trans fatty acids that not only raise LDL but also lower HDL. They also contribute to inflammation in the arteries, another risk factor for heart disease. Those trans fatty acids also occur in the oils used in fast-food restaurants for deep-frying, especially when the oil is repeatedly heated.

That's it. That's all you need to watch for in the way of fats. We've learned that virtually all other fats are either good for your heart or are neutral in their effects. That's particularly true for the omega-3 fatty acids found in fish. While we want to choose lean cuts of beef, opt for the oiliest fish including salmon, herring and sardines. The omega-3 fatty acids protect the heart by limiting formation of blood clots, reducing arterial inflammation and lowering both triglycerides and blood pressure. More about that on page 185.

Until the nineties, we thought it was best to cut right back on nuts of all sorts, as they are quite high in fat. But research has now documented that nuts are actually good for your heart. In fact, those who snack on nuts regularly, even daily, are more protected against heart disease than those who eat no nuts. Nuts of all kinds – almonds, walnuts, pecans, cashews, peanuts and peanut butter – have little saturated fat. Instead they are rich in polyunsaturated fat that improves cholesterol levels.

When shopping for margarine, look for soft types sold in tubs rather than hard types. But read the label to choose brands low in saturated fats, and especially with the lowest overall fat content, that contain plant sterols (phytosterols) clinically proven to lower cholesterol. Two to three servings daily, about what you'd put on that number of slices of bread, provides sufficient amounts of sterols to produce a significant lowering of both total and LDL cholesterol in a matter of weeks when consumed daily.

I personally use and enjoy a wide variety of oils. Olive oil is great for sautéing certain foods, and is a staple in the Mediterranean diet that's best for blood pressure control. Rapeseed oil is also rich in monounsaturated fatty acids that help lower cholesterol when used to replace saturated fats. I like walnut oil for salads, mixed with raspberry vinegar as a dressing. Peanut oil gives oriental food a wonderful taste. Other oils, including soya, safflower and corn oils are low in saturates and high in polyunsaturated fatty acids.

Although all healthy diets should include a spectrum of fruits and vegetables – at the very least, five servings daily – and wholegrain breads and cereals, cutting back too much on animal protein and healthy fats and oils can tip the scales in the wrong direction. A very low-fat diet that's also low in protein is not only boring and not very tasty but also tends to raise levels of triglycerides and to lower protective HDL. Again, go for lean cuts of meats and poultry, lots of fish and seafood, fat-free or low-fat dairy foods, and oils such as olive and rapeseed – limited only by calories if you eat too much.

Numerous studies have determined that a diet low in saturated and trans fats can typically reduce cholesterol levels by 5 to 8 per cent. That's a good start, of course, but many men and women need to do more. As noted, however, cutting back too much on fat and protein and eating a diet heavily dominated by plant-based foods may lower total and LDL cholesterol, but HDL and triglycerides will be adversely affected. Remember that the ratio of total to HDL cholesterol is a better predictor of heart disease risk than either total or LDL cholesterol.

You can improve that ratio by including foods in your diet that are rich in soluble fibre. Foods including oat meal (porridge) and oat bran, beans and peas of all sorts such as chickpeas and kidney beans, as well as figs and barley, are all great sources of soluble fibre. Regularly including them in your diet can bring your LDL cholesterol down by another 5 per cent or more while not lowering HDL cholesterol at all. And, as a special bonus, research has shown that a diet rich in soluble fibre also promotes lower blood pressure.

Blocking cholesterol from the foods you eat

Let's say that you're right on the border between a healthy and dangerous cholesterol level. A 10 per cent reduction might be all you need. Well, nature has provided a great solution by way of the plant world's equivalent of cholesterol itself.

Just as all animal tissue and foods contain cholesterol, needed for life itself, all plants have phytosterols, plant sterols. The molecular structures of cholesterol and phytosterols are virtually identical. Because they are so similar, the human body cannot tell the difference.

As such, phytosterols are readily accepted into the receptor sites of specialised cells called micelles that transport cholesterol directly into the bloodstream from the digestive tract. Those micelles are located in the first third of the small intestine. Early research showed that only a limited amount of cholesterol could be transported into the blood from the gastrointestinal (GI) tract at a time.

Give those receptor sites phytosterols and they accept them as though they were cholesterol, thus blocking cholesterol itself. The trick, then, is to take concentrated phytosterols in tablet form at the beginning of a meal, especially meals containing animal foods that have cholesterol. Bear in mind that all animal foods have essentially the same amount of cholesterol whether lean or fatty; in fact, chicken breast has more than beef.

Some foods, of course, have more cholesterol than others. Eggs, organic meats and prawns are particularly cholesterol-rich. For about ten years, I never ate a single egg yolk. Since discovering how well the phytosterols work, I now enjoy eggs in all forms regularly and my cholesterol tests have never been better. I just swallow a couple of tablets at the start of the meal.

So, one mode of action for phytosterols is to inhibit or completely block absorption of dietary cholesterol into the bloodstream. But they work in another, entirely different, way as well. That's by preventing the recycling of bile, made from cholesterol, following a meal. Phytosterols attach to the bile, which is then eliminated in the bowel movement. That's why taking plant sterols improves cholesterol levels even when used before meals that have little or no cholesterol at all.

Between those two modes of action, including phytosterols on a regular, daily basis will lower your total cholesterol by about 10 per cent and your LDL by up to 14 per cent, while not reducing HDL at all. The result is a much improved ratio and decreased risk of developing or progressing heart disease.

Sound too good to be true? More than 1,200 research studies, conducted at top medical centres around the world and published in the most prestigious medical journals, document both the safety and efficacy of phytosterols in cholesterol control. They are completely safe not only because they are naturally found in plants but also because they never enter the bloodstream. After blocking the receptor micelles for probably one to two hours, they are rejected owing to the slight difference in molecular structure and are eliminated by the body. Even children and pregnant women can take them without fear.

Phytosterol supplement tablets are widely available. But I am aware of only one brand formulated for immediate release. Why is that important? Most tablets take 20 to 30 minutes to dissolve in the stomach before they can release their plant sterols to block cholesterol. Therefore one must either time swallowing the tablets or accept the fact that cholesterol will compete with the phytosterol at the receptor sites in the digestive tract. Some of the cholesterol will get into the bloodstream. But if the phytosterol is immediately released it goes straight to those receptor micelles and leaves no room for cholesterol so that one needn't time the dose and will get a better cholesterol improvement.

The immediate-release formulation of phytosterols is made by Endurance Products Company, based outside of Portland, Oregon. Their website is www.endur.com. Click on Customer Service, International Orders. That's the same company that makes the best formulation of my favourite method of cholesterol control, niacin.

Niacin – your heart's best friend

Niacin is a vitamin, B3, but when taken in doses larger than needed for nutrition it is the best agent in the world for cholesterol control. Not even the prescription drugs come close. That's because niacin affects the entire spectrum in the lipid panel.

Total and LDL cholesterol levels fall by an average of 20 to 40 per cent. This fall has been documented again and again at major medical centres worldwide.

Protective levels of the good HDL cholesterol rise. Improvements in HDL occur in both patients with raised and normal triglycerides, whereas the drug gemfibrozil, for example, works only when triglycerides are raised. Often HDL improvements can be made even with niacin doses as low as 500mg, as documented by doctors in Israel and elsewhere. At the Mayo Clinic, in Rochester, Minnesota, 63 participants in a cardiac rehabilitation programme who had low HDL levels experienced an average 18 per cent increase with niacin. Doctors at the Ochsner Clinic, in New Orleans, achieved a 32 per cent HDL improvement.

Triglyceride measurements fall precipitously with niacin. The higher the initial levels, the greater the response. In a study supported by the National Institutes of Health in the US, triglycerides fell on average by 52 per cent. Other studies show 15 to 30 per cent reductions or higher, depending on the dose.

And only niacin offers benefits in regard to newly determined, independent risk factors for development and progression of heart disease and incidence of heart attack and stroke. It lowers levels of a particularly nasty variant of LDL termed lipoprotein (a). The vitamin improves the balance of the hormone-like substances called prostaglandins, with the detrimental thromboxane falling and the protective prostacycline going up. Activity of blood platelets, cells involved in the clotting process, was decreased, resulting in fewer clots that can lead to heart attacks.

Doctors now recognise that small, dense particles of LDL cholesterol are more dangerous than larger, buoyant particles. Niacin causes a shift from small, dense LDL to large, buoyant particles. No prescription drug can do that!

Finally, niacin lowers levels of inflammation in the arteries. As total and LDL cholesterol fall along with lipoprotein (a), HDL goes up, and other benefits are achieved, measurements of inflammation decrease.

Niacin can be used either alone, which, for most men and women seeking cholesterol control, is enough, or in combination with the statin drugs. In fact, research at the University of Washington and elsewhere proves that the combination represents the state-of-the-art approach to aggressive cholesterol control, completely stopping progression of heart disease and even reversing blockage of the arteries.

In view of the current medical consensus that LDL cholesterol levels should be as low as possible, especially for those with a personal or family history of heart disease, and that all aspects of the lipid profile should be controlled as well, niacin is essential. One could also make a strong case for saying that a person at risk of heart attack or stroke is not being effectively treated if he or she is not taking niacin as part of the total heart health regimen.

Niacin benefits heart health when used at doses significantly higher than when the vitamin is viewed in nutritional terms. It works its wonders in the liver, the principal site of cholesterol manufacture by the body. As such, niacin usage should be monitored by one's doctor. Regular tests will determine not only cholesterol levels but also the health of the liver. Be sure to discuss this with your doctor. He or she will certainly be aware just how well niacin works as your heart's best friend. If not, point him or her to the references cited at the end of this book.

Historically, the biggest problem with niacin was the virtual certainty of flushing of the skin. This has been likened to the hot flushes experienced by women going through menopause. My comparison is to rolling around in the sand after getting a nasty sunburn. Not very pleasant. But that's history.

There are now sustained-release formulations of niacin that practically eliminate flushing by allowing niacin to enter the bloodstream gradually. The best of these is made by the Endurance Products Company. Their product, Endur-acin, has been extensively clinically tested and evaluated at the University of Minnesota and elsewhere for both safety and efficacy. It is recommended by doctors throughout the US, including Dr Thomas Pickering, a highly recognised authority in blood pressure control and hypertension at the Cornell Medical Center in New York. Look for it at www.endur.com. Click on Customer Service, International Orders. Your heart will thank you for it!

The dose determined to be the safest and most effective is one 500mg tablet of Endur-acin three times daily for a total of 1,500mg a day. That's much lower than previously used in medical research with inferior formulations of niacin. Most individuals take it with meals, as a way to remember to take all three tablets daily. But the scheduling is not absolutely important. For example, I take my evening dose at bedtime, when I brush my teeth. What matters is to remember to take it three times a day. To help me remember, I keep some in my car, office, kitchen, attaché and travel cases and golf bag. I know how important niacin is to my heart health – I really believe it's the single most vital thing I did to save my own life – and I don't want to forget to take even one dose. But if you do happen to forget, say, the midday tablet, double up the dose in the evening.

A prescription-only sustained-release niacin, NiaSpan, has been widely promoted to doctors, but the formulation, frankly, is inferior to that of Endur-acin. Readers of mine whose doctors convinced them to switch from Endur-acin to NiaSpan have written to me complaining of flushing and gastric disturbances.

I want you to know that I don't own stock in the Endurance Products Company and that I don't get a cent for recommending Endur-acin. I do so because I believe it is the best niacin formulation in the world, and I want my readers to have the best.

Speaking of the best, please be sure to avoid the worst! There are unscrupulous companies that sell products labelled as 'No-Flush Niacin'. These are either niacinamide, a metabolite of niacin, or inositol hexanicotinate. Neither of these have any effect whatsoever on cholesterol levels. Despite claims to the contrary, neither have been shown to affect cholesterol at all. Niacin breaks down to niacinamide in the body, but only the niacin, not the amide form, has benefit. And the inositol hexanicotinate, simply enough, does not provide any niacin at all, as proven in clinical studies. Please do not believe any internet advertisements or claims made by sales staff in health food stores or elsewhere.

Additional options for cholesterol control

For most men and women, a heart-healthy diet rich in soluble fibre and supplemented with phytosterols and niacin will control cholesterol very nicely. In fact, expect that your doctor will be amazed at your results. But there are other natural approaches as well.

Red yeast rice has been a staple in Chinese medicine and cooking for centuries. It has been clinically proven to reduce LDL cholesterol. That makes sense since red yeast rice is a natural source of the statin drug lovastatin, though products contain a much lower level of the substance. It's available in pharmacies and health food stores.

Policosanol was first researched by doctors in Cuba. It is derived from the waxy outer coating of sugar cane, which is grown extensively in that country. Studies showed its effectiveness to be equal to that of low doses of prescription statin drugs. Very little research, however, has been done outside of Cuba, and results of that research have never been published in any major medical journal. It appears, none-theless, to be an effective tool in cholesterol control. The problem, sadly, is finding a product that actually provides 20mg per dose of good-quality policosanol. There is little uniformity among products sold.

Prescription drugs

In 1984, when I began my own fight against heart disease in general and cholesterol in particular, there were only two prescription drugs available. These were in the class known as bile-sequestering resins, which worked by binding to bile from the digestive tract and removing it from the body, causing cholesterol to be drawn from the bloodstream to make more.

Both brands of those resin drugs were particularly nasty to take. Imagine pouring foul-tasting and smelling sand into a glass of water or juice, swirling it into a slurry, and gulping it down before it could settle out. Now do that two, three, even four times daily as prescribed.

I wanted no part of them, and went on to develop the natural alternative programme of oat bran and niacin along with a low-fat diet. (Some would say that niacin, actually, is a drug since it works very differently in large doses than it would as a nutrient. And, as stated, niacin calls for medical supervision taken in those large doses.)

The next class of drugs that came along were the so-called fibrate derivatives including gemfibrozil (Lopid). They did an adequate job of reducing triglycerides and raising HDL, but achieved only marginal LDL improvements. And niacin did a better job on all fronts, though at the time doctors thought huge doses, up to 8g per day, were needed and only the standard, crystalline niacin was available. The flushing and gastric disturbances made patient compliance understandably poor. Endur-acin, of course, ended those problems.

Next we come to the modern class of prescribed cholesterol-lowering drugs, the statins. These are the drugs seen frequently on TV and in magazine advertisements. The first of this class, lovastatin (Mevacor), got US Food and Drug Administration (FDA) clearance in the US in August of 1987. Including lovastatin, there are currently six statin drugs on the market, including simvastatin (Zocor), pravastatin sodium (Lipostat), fluvastatin (Lescol), atorvastatin (Lipitor), and rosuvastatin (Crestor). A seventh statin, cerivastatin (Baycol), was taken off the market following drug-related deaths.

All these drugs have the same mode of action. They are HMG co-A reductase inhibitors. Simply stated, they inhibit the liver's production of an enzyme essential to the manufacture of cholesterol. These are very powerful drugs, the most potent of which are atorvastatin and rosuvastatin, capable of reducing cholesterol, especially LDL, by 50 per cent or more.

In all honesty, these drugs appear to be relatively safe as a class. They have been used for two decades, prescribed to many millions of men and women around the world. And studies have demonstrated that they can prevent heart attacks and strokes and save lives by dramatically reducing cholesterol. Obviously there were terrible problems with cerivastatin (Baycol). And the British medical journal *The Lancet* has asked for a recall of rosuvastatin (Crestor), citing poor research data and potential side effects involving the liver and kidneys and muscle damage. Consumer advocates in the US have also called for FDA to reverse its approval.

Those taking statin drugs should have regular liver function tests, typically every six months or so. Those tests measure levels of liver enzymes. It's also important to report any muscle aches or weakness when taking these drugs, as they might be early signs of muscle damage that could become severe. Permanent deterioration of muscle tissue, termed rhabdomyolysis, is an infrequent, but very real, adverse reaction. Many doctors believe such problems can be avoided by limiting the dose. And if greater cholesterol reduction than that achieved at a low dose is required, combination therapy can help patients reach their goals.

Research at the University of California at Davis (UC Davis) indicates that the side effects of the statin drugs may be due to depletion of a substance naturally produced by the body called co-enzyme Q10 or simply Q10. It turns out that the very same enzyme needed to make cholesterol in the liver is necessary for the production of Q10.

Q10 is found throughout the body, literally in all tissues. Another name for it is ubiquinone, indicating that it is ubiquitous – everywhere – in the body. It is involved in energy production within muscle cells. As we age, Q10 production declines. And statin drugs further deplete the body's Q10 resources. Based on their preliminary, currently unpublished investigations, the UC Davis researchers suggest that all patients taking a statin drug take Q10 supplements as a safeguard against muscle damage. They recommend doses from 150mg to 600mg, depending on the dose of statin drugs taken.

Statin users should also be aware of a little known food-drug interaction involving grapefruit. Several studies have come to the same conclusion. Grapefruit and grapefruit juice vastly increase the amount of statin drug in the blood – by as much as 12-fold. Although grapefruit is an excellent food and a great source of vitamin C, statin users should probably avoid it.

While statin drugs can dramatically lower LDL cholesterol, they do very little to raise HDL or to lower triglycerides or lipoprotein (a) or to improve the other parameters that I explained earlier that niacin influences beneficially. There's no doubt in my mind that niacin is the better choice.

But some men and women have extremely high levels of LDL. For such patients, the best approach would be a combination of a low dose of a statin drug and niacin. That would be particularly advisable if the person has already experienced a heart attack or stroke or has had heart bypass surgery or angioplasty (blood vessel surgery). Such individuals need to get their LDL as low as possible. And the best way to achieve that is with the statin/niacin combination. If you're in that position, and your doctor baulks at the idea of niacin, ask him or her to look at the medical literature. Otherwise, find another doctor.

In conclusion

Twenty-five years ago, few people had even heard of cholesterol, let alone knew what it was. Today it's a household word. As one of the 'Big Three' risk factors for cardiovascular disease, it's something that just has to be controlled. Doing so is easier and more effective than ever before. And the cholesterol/blood pressure connection has been well established.

Chapter 12

Eating Your Way Out of the Pressure Cooker

During the early 1950s, when I was eight or nine years old hanging around the kitchen asking my mother questions about foods and cooking, and really getting into it at that early age, a researcher at the University of Minnesota was thinking about food, lifestyle and health. Dr Ancel Keys, working with scientists around the world, launched one of the most provocative and influential investigations ever. The Seven Countries Study led to us focusing on the fact that how we live and what we eat greatly influences our health. And pestering my mum around the kitchen led to a lifelong love of food and cooking.

Rates of heart disease in Italy, Greece and Japan, where diets low in animal fats and high in fruits, vegetables, seafood and oils predominated, were extremely low. But where dietary and lifestyle patterns were reversed, in Yugoslavia, Finland, the Netherlands and the United States, incidence of heart disease soared. Careful research continued through the 1960s and 1970s. Now, in the twenty-first century, we have pretty much worked out the details as to how to keep our hearts and bodies healthy and to prevent cardiovascular disease in general and heart attacks and strokes in particular.

We live in a much smaller world today, in a cultural sense. Crete, a Greek island where those early studies were done, now has a McDonald's and other fast-food restaurants, and the traditional Mediterranean diet is sadly on the wane. Similar changes have occurred in Japan and Italy, as well as in France, another country where healthy eating and active lifestyle dominated in the past. Not surprisingly, those who have traded olive oil for butter and soups and fresh fish for cheeseburgers have seen their cholesterol and blood pressure levels rise. The World Health Organization calculates that 600 million men and women in the world now have hypertension and that three million die from it each year.

Conversely, when the traditionally healthy food choices from the Mediterranean and Asia replace poor eating habits in the US and elsewhere in the world, health improves. And the good news is that making those sorts of changes does not mean living a life of deprivation. Nor does it mean completely eliminating our favourite regional foods that we've grown up with, wherever we happen to live.

Before getting much further into the science behind heart-healthy nutrition, and eating patterns known to reduce blood pressure, I want to make it perfectly clear that I love food as much as ever, if not even more. I'm definitely not one of the 'Food Police' who take all the joy out of eating. To me, food is a gift to be celebrated not just once in a while but every day! What I've learned is to marry the nutritious and the delicious. In the pages to come, I'll make your mouth water as I show you ways to keep both your heart and your taste buds happy.

Scientific proof of the benefits of heart-healthy eating

You'd think that it wouldn't take thousands of doctors, scientists and nutritionists all over the world to figure out how and what to eat to stay healthy. After all, grandma said, 'Eat your fruits and vegetables.' And, of course, she was absolutely right. But there's more to it than that. Grandma quite likely kept a jar filled with pork fat to use for cooking, like mine did, and my mother as well.

And what about those tales told in every family about Grandad Joe or Uncle Peter who ate bacon and eggs every morning, hated fruit and vegetables, and who demanded meat and potatoes for dinner seven days a week. 'They lived into their nineties, and never had a problem.' Sure. And there certainly are those who smoke cigarettes all their lives without getting lung cancer or emphysema. But those people are the exception to what we now know is the rule.

When I began my career as a medical journalist in the 1960s, many doctors smoked cigarettes. That's not true any more. You have to look long and hard to find a doctor who smokes.

Take a look around you, as my wife Dawn and I did one time when on a sea cruise around the coast of Mexico. We saw a lot of fat people and we saw a lot of old people. But we couldn't spot one person who was both old and fat. You don't have to be a scientist to figure out why. Obese people don't live long.

But it's more than just living long. Quality of life is as important, or more so, than longevity. As the old saying goes, when you have your health you have everything. And in-depth research studies have shown us that you can eat your way to good health. You don't really need the details, but here is some of the proof of the proverbial pudding.

When doctors came to the realisation that fat was associated with cholesterol levels, they threw the baby out with the bathwater, recommending a diet that was low in all fat, not just the saturated fats in meats, dairy products and tropical oils. Yes, when men and women followed that diet, levels of their 'bad' LDL cholesterol came down. But so did the 'good' HDL that protects the heart. And amounts of an independently harmful blood fat, triglycerides, went up. For all their efforts, after giving up a lot of the foods they enjoyed, such people were actually worse off than before.

Today, we know that only two fats hurt the heart. In addition to the saturated fats, trans fatty acids formed by partial hydrogenation of otherwise healthy oils such as soya or sunflower are culprits. They're even worse than saturated fats, in that they lower levels of both LDL and HDL. You find them in processed, pre-packed foods such as bakery products and deep-fried foods in restaurants. All other fats and oils are either beneficial or neutral in their effects on heart health. But, especially in the case of those nasty trans fats, it took decades to learn this, through painstaking research projects all over the world.

Researchers from Denmark collaborated with doctors at the University of Wollongong, in New South Wales, Australia, to determine the effects of saturated, monounsaturated and omega-3 fatty acids on blood pressure in healthy subjects. They found that decreasing saturates and increasing unsaturates led to decreased blood pressure, but that the benefit disappeared when subjects consumed a diet high in fat, 37 per cent of total calories. So, as is so often the case, moderation is the winning ticket.

The same goes for protein. Harvard University investigators have determined that we need a healthy balance of fats, carbohydrates and protein. Not only will adequate amounts of protein provide a greater and more long-lasting feeling of fullness following a meal but also a nice blood pressure lowering in those not currently eating enough. The Harvard scientists recommend a larger daily protein intake than previously believed to be optimal, 25 per cent rather than 15 per cent of calories.

It's no wonder that men and women get frustrated when dietary recommendations change. But the scientific process takes time. The good news is that, while some little bits of tweaking of dietary advice might still happen in the future, we've pretty much got it nailed when it comes to knowing what to eat and what not to eat to keep our hearts healthy.

The Lyon Diet Heart Study gave us the first solid proof of the benefits of the Mediterranean diet in reducing heart disease. French researchers compared that diet, rich in olive oil, nuts, olives, avocados and seafood, with the kind of diet typically prescribed by cardiologists in the UK, US and elsewhere that cut right back on fat, while replacing those calories with carbohydrates. Subjects were patients who had suffered a heart attack within the past six months.

Benefits of the Mediterranean diet started showing up after only a year. And after 27 months, patients on that dietary programme had a significantly lower rate of subsequent heart attack, other heart problems and death. A follow-up analysis nearly four years later demonstrated the long-term advantages. Imagine that enjoying a diet rich in olive oil and other delicious foods actually saved lives!

Italian doctors in the GISSI-Preventione Study had the same happy results when they tried the Mediterranean diet, this time supplemented with omega-3 fatty acids, with heart attack patients. After three and a half years, rates of non-fatal heart attack, stroke and death were down substantially.

The Lyon and GISSI-Preventione studies are particularly noteworthy because their subjects already had heart disease severe enough to have caused heart attacks. If those approaches worked for men and women already suffering heart disease, think what they can do for you!

For example, doctors at the University of Minnesota worked with more than 4,300 healthy young men and women who were aged between 18 and 30 years old at the start of the study and monitored them for 15 years. Those eating the most fruits and vegetables in their diets, as compared with meat and potatoes, had the lowest rate of developing raised blood pressure. But that doesn't mean they gorged on those plant foods. The participants were divided into five groups based on fruit and vegetable consumption, from lowest to highest. Compared with the lowest intake, those in the second lowest to the highest intake had 27 to 36 per cent less likelihood of BPs rising to at least 135/85. So even a little extra effort along these lines can provide a big payoff.

The biggest of all the studies carried out thus far involves the DASH diet, standing for Dietary Approaches to Stop Hypertension, and was begun in the mid-1990s. It was a major undertaking of the US National Institutes of Health, with 459 men and women participating as volunteers in several medical centres around the world. The DASH diet includes lots of fruits, vegetables, wholegrains, seafood and fat-free and low-fat dairy products.

The diet worked. Blood pressure fell by an average of 5.5 systolic and 3 diastolic. Black people responded with drops of 6.9 and 3.3. In those with blood pressure readings higher than 140/90, results were even better, with numbers falling by 11.4 and 5.5 respectively. Cholesterol levels were also improved by 7 per cent.

Medical researchers wondered whether a high-carbohydrate, low-fat diet or a diet higher in monounsaturated fats would be better for diabetic patients. The high-carb, low-fat diet actually tended to raise systolic and diastolic blood pressure by 6 and 7 mmHg, respectively, for the 42 subjects with type 2 diabetes, while the higher fat diet lowered both systolic and diastolic BP by three to four points after a 14-week period.

Why does this sort of diet work so well? One theory is that a diet rich in fruits, vegetables and fat-free and low-fat dairy foods might work as a natural diuretic, much like certain drugs prescribed for lowering blood pressure. Those medications have been used to fight hypertension for decades. It's still unknown whether the blood pressure effects resulting from the diet are a consequence of a specific food or foods or a combination of all of them. The diet is rich in potassium and calcium, both of which help eliminate sodium from the body in the urine. But apparently there's more to it than those two minerals, since taking supplements doesn't yield as strong a result.

Another reason, some scientists believe, might be the effect of plant protein as compared with animal protein. The INTERMAP study involved 4,680 men and women from the US, UK, Japan and China, representing diverse populations. Consumption of animal protein didn't affect blood pressure. But plant protein intake was significantly correlated with lower BP.

So many studies have shown enormous benefits in consuming omega-3 fatty acids from both fish and supplements. They have a powerful influence on improving blood pressure, and have many other advantages for heart health.

But, hey, who really cares why these sorts of diets work? The important thing is that they work!

At least one study has shown that patients with mildly raised blood pressure can bring levels down with this diet alone. And for those needing prescription drugs, the diet can lower the doses required. But the best news is that combining this dietary approach, modified to suit your personal tastes and food preferences, along with the newly proven supplements detailed in this book, eliminates the need for prescription drugs for all but the most severe cases of hypertension.

Whichever part or parts of the diet provide the heart-saving benefits, we know for sure that fruits and vegetables are essential, and have been proven to slash the risk of stroke. Doctors in Australia and England, reporting in the medical journal *The Lancet*, combined the data from multiple studies involving more than a quarter of a million subjects over a course of 13 years on average. Compared with those who ate less than three servings of fruit and vegetables daily, men and women who consumed three to five had 11 per cent less risk of stroke, and those who gobbled more than five servings saw their stroke risk tumble by 26 per cent.

Combining wise dietary choices with other lifestyle improvements including cigarette cessation and exercise and weight control pay off even higher dividends. In an on-going US study involving thousands of nurses conducted through Harvard University, scientists have calculated that fully 82 per cent of heart disease events could potentially be prevented. For non-smokers, further lifestyle modifications could slash the risk by 74 per cent. Studies around the globe have demonstrated similar protection.

So what, exactly, does the Mediterranean diet consist of and how is it different from the average Western diet? Actually, it's more a matter of complete lifestyle that begins with regular physical activity and wine in moderation (although other forms of alcoholic beverages probably provide similar if not identical protection – see pages 147–8). Daily foods include eight servings of wholegrain breads and cereals, six servings of vegetables, three of fruit, two of dairy foods, and just about all the olive oil one would want short of gaining weight. On a weekly basis, there would be five to six servings of fish and seafood, four of poultry, three to four of olives, nuts, and beans, three of potatoes, three eggs and three desserts. A strict Mediterranean diet would allow only four servings of red meat, though, as we'll see, there's room for variations and modifications to suit one's own tastes and preferences.

But what about those fruits and vegetables? Aren't the amounts recommended by advocates of the Mediterranean diet and eaten by people in Greece, Spain, Italy and elsewhere in that part of the world huge? Not really, when you take a closer look at just what a serving size is.

An average serving of fruit is 80g and that of vegetables 77g. That would be one average apple, half a banana, 100ml of apple sauce, two tablespoons of raisins or a 200ml glass of fruit juice. A serving of cooked vegetables is 75g. For raw veggies, it's 150g or a glass of tomato, carrot or other vegetable juice.

How might that fit into an average day? For breakfast you might start with a glass of juice. You could then slice half a banana into your cereal or add 40g of blueberries or other fruit. At your mid-morning and mid-afternoon break, you could replace the coffee and doughnut with a glass of juice or a piece of fruit, at least two or three days a week. For snacks, keep a ready supply of dried fruits at home, in the car, and where you work.

Most of us are far too busy to do much in the way of making lunch. And, without planning, that can mean urgent hunger that's satisfied with high-calorie, high-fat, low-nutrient fast food. Here's a suggestion for something faster: soup. A nice steaming bowl is extremely satisfying and remarkably soothing at midday. Choose chicken and vegetable, minestrone, lentil, split pea, beef and barley, the list goes on. Either order a bowl at a restaurant or bring some from home and heat it up in a microwave. You'll get two or three servings of veggies or even more, in that one meal.

I love salad sandwiches. They're a delicious and convenient way to get a couple of servings of veggies. And I ask for some slices of smoked salmon to be added, not only to get some heart-healthy omega-3 fatty acids but also because I happen to really love that fish.

For the evening meal, get into the habit of putting two or three different vegetables on the plate. Start the meal with a nice salad or a cup of soup. Then, for evening snacks, more fruit.

What about cost? One doctor wrote a letter to *The Lancet* pointing out that in Scotland, 48 per cent of the population eat fresh fruit once a week or less and 41 per cent eat green vegetables once a week or less. He suggested that perhaps it was a matter of economics. But that's just not true. First, at least in most parts of the world, seasonal fruits and vegetables are inexpensive. Second, when fresh may not be available, one can use frozen produce that will provide virtually identical nutritional value. Actually, studies have demonstrated that frozen fruits and vegetables can be higher in nutrients than their fresh counterparts since they are fast frozen almost immediately after harvest, while fresh produce may be days old by the time fruits and vegetables are picked, boxed, shipped and on the shelf.

For most people, the problem with fruits and vegetables, to be perfectly honest, is that they are boring. Eating steamed vegetables every night would take the dedication of a monk. Fruit can be more interesting if one aims for variety. But even then, you eventually run out of different kinds. So how do those people in the Mediterranean and elsewhere eat so much plant food? They're much more creative. That's why I've provided a lot of ideas about preparation in the recipe section, Chapter 17. And consider some perhaps unusual choices. Pomegranates have been a healthy part of the diets in the Middle East and the Mediterranean for centuries. Several recent studies have demonstrated their protective benefits against heart disease and raised blood pressure. The crunchy ruby-red seeds are filled to bursting with juicy flavour and nutrients including vitamin C and potassium. Enjoy them as a snack or as colourful and different additions in salads.

When my children were little, I wanted to instil a love of fruits and veggies. But kids aren't any different from adults. They have to be tempted. Offer a child – or an adult – a bowl of apples or pears or peaches and you won't see much excitement.

So when Ross and Jenny came home from school, looking for a snack, I came up with some tempting treats. Instead of a whole apple, I sliced that apple and used raisins to make faces. Pretty simple. Other times I'd slice a variety of fruits and offer them on a plate with some fruit-flavoured yogurt as a dip. When I had the time and wanted to be creative, I shaped red and green peppers to look like 'palm fronds' when added to the 'trunks' of longitudinally sliced carrots, perhaps with a 'bush' of broccoli, and a 'pond' of low-fat salad dressing on a plate. Mothers in the neighbourhood began to wonder why their kids wanted to come to our house after school! Yup, I was 'Mr Mum'. And I loved it.

Again, adults aren't much different from children. Take the time to do similar preparation for yourself and you'll enjoy those snacks a whole lot more.

Chocolate's healthy side

In Woody Allen's comedy film *Sleeper*, doctors in the distant future comment on how hot fudge sundaes were eventually found to be a 'health food'. In a turn suggesting that life does, in fact, sometimes imitate art, research for the past decade has focused on the heart-health benefits of dark chocolate.

One such report came from the University of L'Aguila, in Italy, in 2005. Researchers there, in collaboration with doctors at Tufts University, in Boston, found that dark chocolate, thanks to its high content of plant substances called flavonoids, lowered blood pressure nicely. They gave patients 100g of either dark chocolate or white chocolate daily. The dark confection, but not the white, brought systolic BP down by 11.9 mmHg and diastolic BP down 8.5 mmHG. In fact, the darker the chocolate, the greater the level of those beneficial flavonoids.

But eating chocolate every day isn't a realistic approach to blood pressure control. You'd get 580 calories from that 100g bar, along with 45g of fat, 27.5g of which are saturated. Much of the research has been sponsored by the Mars company, based in Chicago, Illinois. While that company has enjoyed expected headlines in the media, the real purpose is to eventually isolate the specific flavonoids, synthesise the chemicals, and make them available perhaps as a prescription drug for blood pressure. That would be a good thing, since such a 'drug' would not be expected to have the adverse effects of drugs on the market now. But it would be years before that product might hit the pharmacy shelves.

In the meantime, we can all reap the benefits of chocolate without the fat and calories. Chocolate is made from cocoa, butter, cocoa butter and sugar. The healthy flavonoids are in the cocoa. So enjoy cocoa in a variety of delicious ways including hot cocoa and the desserts detailed in the recipe section in this chapter. Buy pure cocoa powder, not the instant mixes that also contain sugar and fat, to get the most in the way of both flavonoids and flavour.

Coffee, tea, cola and your heart

How do you start your day? Most men and women get going with a cup of coffee or tea. Your choice may well be having an impact on heart health in general and blood pressure in particular.

An on-going long-term study involving nearly 156,000 nurses that monitors their lifestyles and health provided some insights in 2005. Harvard researchers compared coffee and cola consumption with the nurses' development of hypertension over a 12-year period. Habitual coffee drinking wasn't associated with increased blood pressure, but cola drinks, both diet and regular, were. Digging further into the data, those women consuming the most caffeine, whether from coffee or cola, were at no greater risk than those with the lowest intake. Why, then, might cola pose some risk? That'll be determined, we hope, by further research.

In the meantime, however, it appears that coffee drinkers can breathe a sigh of relief and enjoy their beverage of choice in moderation. Conversely, it might be a good idea to limit cola drinking and perhaps now and then switch to other types of soft drink.

An exception for coffee drinkers came from work done by Swiss investigators, who found that drinking two cups of caffeinated coffee decreases blood flow to the heart during exercise, especially at high altitudes. On a practical level, it seems that one should keep coffee drinking to just one cup before exercise and to avoid it entirely while climbing or hiking in the mountains.

So much for blood pressure, but what about coffee and cholesterol? There have been mixed reports, and many consumers are justifiably confused. It is true that coffee can raise levels of the harmful LDL cholesterol, but only when prepared in the French or Scandinavian styles. Using a French press (*cafetiere*) coffee maker or dumping ground coffee beans into boiling water, it appears, releases two chemicals called diterpenes that are wholly responsible for increased LDL. Filter coffee making, which does not squeeze the grounds or use boiling-hot water, has no ill effects on cholesterol. Decaf drinkers aren't completely out of the woods. If your brew is made from robusta rather than Arabica beans, coffee can, unfortunately, raise LDL counts. Robusta beans, which are less expensive than the Arabica type, are often used in decaf since they are stronger and provide more flavour following the decaffeination process. It may well be worth the small extra expense to opt for buying decaf made with Arabica beans.

If your beverage of choice happens to be tea, smile when taking the next sip. Or you might even consider switching from coffee to tea after reading this. While coffee, at best, does no harm, tea can provide great benefits in terms of heart health. More than a decade of research has shown us that tea drinkers suffer less heart disease. Chinese investigators in Taiwan have quantified those benefits.

They examined the long-term effects of tea drinking on the development of hypertension and found that the more tea consumed, the lower the risk. The doctors recruited more than 1,500 men and women aged 20 years or older who had no history of raised blood pressure levels. They then recorded how much tea they drank and how many developed hypertension. Those drinking 120–599ml of tea daily showed a 46 per cent decrease in risk, as compared with individuals who typically drink less than 120ml a day. The more the better. Those gulping 600ml or more daily cut their risk by a whopping 65 per cent. When they looked at tea consumption over a ten-year, rather than a one-year, period of time the investigators found no additional benefit.

Those nice benefits are restricted to real tea, not herbal types. It doesn't appear to matter whether tea is decaf or regular, but most of the world's tea drinkers consume regular, full-strength tea. On a practical level, bear in mind that tea contains theobromine, the chemical cousin of caffeine, and drinking large quantities can jangle the nerves just as coffee can. Seek moderation in all things.

Fish, supplements and the search for heart-healthy omega-3 fatty acids

Seldom are research findings unequivocal. Usually one can find data to defend one side of a debate or the other. Omega-3 fatty acids are the exception to the rule. The more scientists investigate the way fish oils work in the body, the more benefits they find, with virtually no negatives to report.

Initially, of course, we heard about the Inuit people of Greenland and how they almost never developed heart disease even though they ate large amounts of fat in the form of fish and marine animals. At first glance that appeared paradoxical. Then came the realisation that the fat consumed was a kind of polyunsaturated fatty acid termed omega-3. Think about it: if the fat in cold-water fish were saturated, those fish would be as stiff and hard as a pack of butter in the refrigerator.

Next was a long-term study of workers at the Western Electric Company in Chicago, hinting that fish lovers enjoyed protection against heart disease. The risk of fatal heart attack was slashed by a third with just this one lifestyle factor. A similar investigation that examined the habits of tens of thousands of male doctors revealed that those who ate fish at least once a week had half the risk of sudden cardiac death.

The list of research studies goes on and on, all with favourable results. We know now that the major fish oils, eicosapentaenoic acid (EPA) and docosahexaenoic acid (DHA), work in a number of wonderful ways. These omega-3 fatty acids reduce the formation of blood clots and raise levels of the protective HDL cholesterol while dramatically lowering triglycerides. They help prevent heart rhythm disturbances and lower heart rates. Because heart rate is associated with risk of sudden death, this association may explain at least partially the lower risk of sudden death among those who regularly eat fish.

A fairly new observation shows the ability of omega-3s to lower blood pressure. It appears to do so by reducing resistance to surges of blood flow in the arteries. That, in turn, improves performance of the left ventricle of the heart, the muscular pump. What we have, as a result, is healthier arteries that are less stiff and more flexible and a more powerful heart muscle, both these factors improve blood flow and hence reduce blood pressure.

Both fish itself and fish oil supplements providing omega-3 fatty acids EPA and DHA have been clinically documented to yield these benefits for the heart and vascular system. It turns out that even small amounts of fish, especially the fatty, cold-water fish including salmon, herring, sardines and mackerel, do the trick. One needn't eat fish daily, giving up all meats. The Food Standards Agency recommends having two fish meals weekly – at least one an oily fish. That's solidly backed up in the medical literature.

I happen to be one of those lucky guys who really loves fish. In restaurants, I most frequently order salmon, not just because it's 'good for me' but because I simply enjoy it, whether grilled, roasted, blackened or poached. For a little snack to tide me over before dinner I'll have herring, either pickled or creamed, on wholewheat crackers. Smoked salmon on a bagel with a dab of low-fat cream cheese? That's heaven to me!

But not everyone likes, much less loves, fish. For them, supplements are the answer. After many years of experimentation most authorities now agree on the optimal dose. If buying fish oil capsules, aim for 3g daily. You can also get EPA and DHA in a concentrated ethyl ester form, in which case you need only 1g a day. Those using omega-3 supplements to reduce very high levels of triglycerides will require 3.5g daily; that dose is considered 'pharmacologic', acting like a drug, and should be taken under medical supervision.

You may hear about getting omega-3s from plant sources, especially flaxseed and flaxseed oil but also including soya, rapeseed and walnut oils, and various kinds of nuts. All those foods contain a far less potent form of the beneficial fatty acids called alpha-linolenic acid (ALA). You may even see ALA supplements on sale in health food stores and pharmacies. But only a fraction, a small fraction, of ALA is converted by the body into EPA and DHA. Stick with the fish oils or the concentrated ethyl ester supplements.

There is only one broad contraindication. Patients taking the potent blood-thinning drug warfarin by prescription from their doctors should not, under any circumstances, take omega-3 supplements. In fact, if you take those drugs discuss with your doctor what is a safe consumption of fish.

Omega-3 fatty acid content of fish in grams/100g serving

Fish	Amount	Fish	Amount
Sardines (Norway)	5.1	Tuna steaks	1.3
Sockeye salmon	2.7	Halibut	1.3
Mackerel (Atlantic)	2.5	Mackerel (Pacific)	1.1
King salmon	1.9	Sea bass	0.8
Herring	1.7	Tinned tuna	0.6

But what about mercury contamination of fish? It's true that mercury, a heavy metal, becomes concentrated in the fatty tissues of fish. That's particularly true for swordfish and shark, all of which have one part per million or more. Consumption of these fish should be limited to one portion per week for men and older women and avoided altogether by children and women of childbearing age. But, as reported in the 28 November 2002 issue of the *New England Journal of Medicine*, many if not most fish do not have appreciable amounts. Fresh and frozen tuna have 0.32 parts per million (ppm) and tinned tuna drops down to 0.17 ppm. Pollack has 0.20 ppm. And in both salmon and shrimp, mercury is not detectable.

Certainly the small amounts of mercury in fish other than those with one or more ppm do not pose a threat, and the benefits to heart health far outweigh any potential risk. Pregnant women and small children, however, should limit consumption of fish varieties higher in the heavy metal. As with all such matters, discuss this with your doctor. Current UK advice is that girls and women of childbearing age (especially if pregnant or breastfeeding) should have a maximum of two portions of oily fish a week. For males and older women the maximum is four portions a week. For tinned tuna there is no limit set for men and older women. But women of childbearing age and especially pregnant/ breastfeeding women should have no more than four tins per week. There is no recommended limit for white fish.

Dietary variations around the world

For the most part, people tend to eat and enjoy the foods they grew up with. It's stating the obvious to say that French people like French food, Italians love Italian dishes, and those living in China prefer not only Chinese food, but specifically the preparations from the province of their birth. Although I really like Chinese food, after a month's stay in that country, I was really tired of it.

I've always thought that those of us who live in the UK, US, Canada, Australia and other countries with a large immigrant population are lucky to have ready access to a wide variety of different cuisines from all over the world. One day it can be Italian, the next day Greek, the day after that Chinese or Thai or Japanese, and on it goes. Moreover, we have our own regional preferences.

Growing up in the American Midwest, I developed and still have a strong affinity for meatloaf with mashed potatoes and gravy. The English invented shepherd's pie, and Englishmen eat it throughout their lives. And Australians love meat pies.

So does it mean that one must abandon those sorts of preferences in order to improve blood pressure readings? Must one eat nothing but Greek food as prepared on the shores of the Mediterranean to follow a 'Mediterranean diet'? Nothing could be further from the truth. One scientific investigation, for example, was titled the Indo-Mediterranean Diet Heart Study, reflecting the influences of Indian cuisine. Next, consider how many very different countries surround the Mediterranean Sea. I'm looking at a map as I write this, noting, beyond the obvious Italy and Greece, countries including Morocco, Algeria, Tunisia, France, Spain, Turkey, Croatia, Albania, and the vast expanse of the Middle Eastern countries such as Egypt, Israel, Syria, Lebanon and others. And don't forget the foods of the Far East, which have also been noted for their heart-healthy qualities. Their national cuisines are very different but have certain things in common: lots of fruits and vegetables, plenty of fish and seafood, poultry, low-fat red meats (including some you might not find in your market, such as goat and water buffalo and camel), wholegrain bread and cereals, and foods and oils rich in monounsaturated fatty acids.

Moreover, and probably most important of all, we can 'tweak' the favoured dishes of our origins to reduce saturated fat and increase monounsaturated fat and vegetables. Yes, even meatloaf, shepherd's pie and meat pies. And olive oil is not necessarily the panacea, the only choice you have. There's also rapeseed oil, which is rich in monounsaturated fats and extremely low in saturated fats. Other oils fill the bill as well. Let me give you one example before starting into a treasure trove of heart-healthy, cholesterol lowering and blood pressure improving recipes. I really enjoy chilli con carne, as do most Americans. But the version I cook today includes two tins of chilli beans instead of one to boost the level of plant protein and soluble fibre, very low-fat minced beef, low-sodium tinned tomatoes and a tin of chilli peppers. I like to sprinkle on grated low-fat cheddar cheese and mellow the chilli with a dollop of low-fat sour cream. Wine just doesn't go well with chilli, so it's always a bottle of beer. Nothing like that was ever served in Greece or Italy, although they have somewhat similar dishes. It has all the heart-healthy attributes of the Mediterranean diet even though its origins lie along the Texas–Mexico border. Assuming that you love food as much as I do, I'm delighted to share some of the Kowalski cookbook with you in the recipes and suggestions I offer in Chapter 17.

Chapter 13

Little Things Mean a Lot (or Not)

We know for certain that blood pressure tends to rise as we get older. Family history plays a big role. High blood pressure, in turn, increases the risk of stroke and heart attack. While there's not much we can do to turn back the hands of time and we can't choose our parents and grandparents, there are a lot of little things that appear to lower BP and risk of cardiovascular disease. Conversely, there are other things, some of which are touted in magazines and health food stores, that have little or no effect or may even raise blood pressure. Perversely, some medications, both over-the-counter and prescription-only, can make BP go up.

Rather than appear to give priority to one or other in this chapter's review of these little things, I've chosen to discuss them in alphabetical order. It's a real pot-pourri of ideas you may or may never have heard of or considered.

Acupuncture

This technique has been used for centuries by Chinese, Japanese and Korean doctors to treat a wide variety of ailments. German researchers looked at the effectiveness of acupuncture in the treatment of high blood pressure and reported their findings at the annual scientific sessions of the American Heart Association in 2005.

They worked with 160 male and female patients aged from 45 to 75 years, all of whom had mild to moderate hypertension. Seventy-eight per cent were taking anti-hypertensive drugs. During a six-week trial, patients were given acupuncture or a sham treatment designed to feel the same as acupuncture.

Of that starting group, 141 patients completed the trial; 72 received acupuncture and 69 received the sham treatment or placebo. Immediately after acupuncture BP fell from an average of 131/81 to 125/78, but the sham treatment had no impact, during a 24-hour period. But when patients were tested three and six months later, there was no residual effect of the acupuncture treatment.

Unless you happen to live with an acupuncture therapist, this doesn't seem to be a practical way to control blood pressure.

Arginine

This amino acid is found naturally in many foods and is available as a supplement. It has received mixed reviews regarding its efficacy in treating hypertension. One study looked at people following an arginine-rich diet, which included a lot of beans and nuts, and who took arginine supplements and found that they did, indeed, reduce systolic blood pressure by an average of 6.2 mmHG and diastolic BP by 5 mmHG compared to the control group.

A small but carefully controlled trial was performed with six diabetes patients who received 3g of arginine hourly for 10 hours. During that period, BP fell by 12 mmHG systolic and 6.2 mmHG diastolic on average. Blood pressure dropped within two hours after starting to take the arginine, but returned to levels prior to arginine after just one hour after stopping the supplement. Now, obviously this sort of treatment isn't very practical. First, the typical arginine supplement capsule contains just 500mg of the amino acid. One would have to take six capsules to reach 3g. Second, patients in that study took the supplements every hour. Third, after the 10-hour trial, when supplementation stopped, BP went right back up.

Discouraging? No. As I detail on page 222, there are now arginine supplements that have been formulated for sustained-release. That not only means one need only take the capsules twice daily but also achieves the same benefit derived from very high doses in a fraction of the amount needed.

Aspirin

Native Americans were peeling the bark off willow trees and drinking a tea brewed from it to ease aches and pains long before Europeans set foot in the New World. Eventually the active ingredient was isolated and identified as acetylsalicylic acid, more commonly known as aspirin. Bayer launched a synthesised aspirin product in 1899 as an anti-inflammatory and painkilling over-the-counter medicine and it quickly became the most widely used agent in the history of medicine.

In 1960, researchers found that aspirin has an 'antiplatelet' activity; it prevents blood cells called platelets from forming clots. Today, the US Food and Drug Administration (FDA) and other regulatory agencies throughout the world approve aspirin to reduce the risk of stroke, for immediate treatment of possible heart attack, and prevention of second heart attacks. And a study of 55,000 patients showed that daily aspirin can prevent a first heart attack in apparently healthy individuals, reducing the risk by 32 per cent.

It's a good thing that no one pharmaceutical manufacturer has an exclusive patent on the stuff or we'd be paying through the nose! Aspirin is one of the cheapest ways to protect our hearts.

Of course, like almost anything else, aspirin can cause problems in certain individuals. It increases the risk of gastrointestinal bleeding and a type of stroke termed haemorrhagic, in which bleeding occurs in the brain. But those adverse reactions are relatively rare, and the risk/benefit ratio is very good.

A meta-analysis of six trials with a total of more than 95,000 men and women was performed and published in 2006. Researchers concluded that aspirin reduced the risk of stroke in women and heart attacks in men. Overall, women taking low doses of aspirin had a 12 per cent lower risk of suffering either a heart attack, stroke or cardiovascular-disease-related death. Post-menopausal women and those who had suffered a previous cardiovascular event experienced the most benefit. Men enjoyed a 14 per cent reduction in risk.

Doctors typically recommend a low-dose 81mg aspirin tablet daily. Some studies have shown effectiveness with 100mg every other day. Taking a coated tablet can reduce the risk of gastric upset and bleeding, but some studies have indicated lesser protection. And preliminary observations show that the optimum time to take one's daily aspirin would be at bedtime rather than in the morning, since it reduces levels of nocturnal blood pressure though not daytime BP.

Breathing

Most of the time humans are 'autobreathers' – we don't give breathing a thought. Well, we should do so. It turns out that when we breathe rapidly and shallowly, as we tend to do much of the day, our blood pressure goes up. Conversely, when we slow down our breathing rate and deliberately breathe deeply both in and out, we can make our blood pressure go down.

If you have decided to purchase a blood pressure monitor, which I discuss in Chapter 2, try this simple test. Walk rapidly to wherever the device is, sit down, start it up, and measure your blood pressure. Jot down the numbers. Then close your eyes and spend two or three minutes concentrating on your breathing. Very deliberately breathe in deeply, feeling your lungs expanding to the fullest. Hold that breath for a bit. Then slowly, slowly let the air out, and, when you think you're completely deflated like a balloon, 'puff' out the last remaining air. Repeat the process. Again, think about the breathing process. Enjoy the process of the air fully inflating your lungs and finally deflating. Now retest your pressure. Almost certainly it'll be lower. Now do another 'session' of deliberate and slow breathing before testing the third time. Your BP will be lower still. Pretty powerful stuff that shows how we have personal control over our bodies.

Is this just a 'parlour trick' that has no lasting effect? If you do it just that one time, yes. But if you make it a habit to take several little 'mini-holidays' a day of deep breathing, eventually you'll see a lasting benefit. In fact, you'll want to get to the point where you breathe fewer times per minute throughout the entire day. How many times per minute do you breathe now? Almost certainly you have no idea unless you make it a point to count your breaths. Do so. Note the number. Then make an effort to breathe fewer times per minute but more fully and deeply. Studies have proved that those who do so will have lower blood pressure.

In fact, there is a device on the market to help you achieve the goal of BP reduction through improved breathing. Aptly termed 'RESPeRATE', the little machine about the size of a paperback book is battery operated and you can take it anywhere. The device automatically analyses your breathing rate and pattern and interactively guides you through a breathing exercise to slow down your breathing from the normal rate of 14 to 18 breaths per minute to the therapeutic zone of less than 10 breaths per minute, with prolonged exhalation as I described above.

At first, breathing returns to 'normal' after each session of RESPeRATE use. But gradually you'll find that your breath-per-minute rate and the depth of your breathing improves. And researchers say the beneficial effects on blood pressure build up to create a lasting BP reduction with regular use.

Clinical studies have shown the device capable of lowering blood pressure by an average of 14 mmHG systolic and 9 mmHG diastolic after eight weeks of routine use consisting of 15 minutes a day three or four times a week. Average reductions, the researchers have found, are greater for older patients and those with higher BPs to begin with. And those reductions would be over and above any from other forms of therapy.

For more information on RESPeRATE go to www.high-blood-pressure-help.com. Can you do it completely on your own without the device? Sure, but optimum benefits will be achieved with the assistance of this little device. There's also the advantage of 'relying' on a machine as though it were a professional psychologist guiding you through breathing sessions. And you'll find this is a wonderful way to deal with stress.

Co-enzyme Q10 (Co-Q10 or Q10)

Q10 is a substance that occurs naturally in virtually all our bodies' tissues, especially in muscle tissue (see page 169). Q10 regulates energy in muscle cells. As we age, amounts decline. For that reason, it has been speculated that taking supplements will improve energy levels. That claim hasn't been well substantiated. But there are other and better reasons to consider supplements.

Statin drugs prescribed to lower cholesterol also lower production of Q10, sometimes to a point of serious deficiency. That's because statin drugs inhibit an enzyme essential for the body's manufacture of both cholesterol and Q10. Medical researchers at the University of California at San Diego believe that the Q10 depletion caused by statin drugs may be responsible for the drug's potential for muscle ache and potential permanent muscle damage. They recommend Q10 supplementation for everyone taking statin drugs.

What about Q10 and blood pressure? Researchers theorise that most hypertensive patients have a significant Q10 deficiency that in turn leads to a deficiency in a naturally occurring pro-vitamin, a substance that 'energises' and maximises the potential of vitamins. At least eight trials looked at the effect of varying doses of Q10 on blood pressure. All showed benefit, though BP reductions varied.

In one trial, 30 patients received 60mg of Q10 twice daily while a control group of 29 other patients got a B-vitamin placebo for eight weeks. The Q10 group had a very nice 16-point drop in systolic BP and a 9-point fall in diastolic pressure. They also saw a reduction in triglycerides, blood sugar and insulin, and increases in HDL and serum levels of vitamins A, C and E. The B-vitamin placebo control group saw only an increase in vitamin C in the blood.

Another study examined the effects of Q10 on what's called isolated systolic hypertension in which only the systolic, not the diastolic, pressure is raised. A group of 46 men and 37 women received either 60mg of Q10 or a placebo daily for 12 weeks. Those taking the Q10 saw a reduction in systolic blood pressure from 10.5 mmHG to a whopping 25.1 mmHG, with an average reduction of 17.8. That's wonderful, but not all studies have shown such dramatic improvements.

Part of the reason for the variance in effectiveness of Q10 may come down to whether a person has a low level of the substance in the tissues and bloodstream to begin with. One could take a test to measure Q10 levels. Or one could simply undertake a two- or three-month trial to see what sort of benefit it might provide. Certainly there are no possible downsides to Q10 supplements, and one might note improvements in energy as well as reduced blood pressure. It might work for you and it might not, but there's no reason not to try it.

Eye tests

Now what could eye tests possibly have to do with blood pressure, you might reasonably ask. Well, it turns out that the eyes may be the window through which to look for potential future hypertension. The little arterioles (tiny arteries) that supply blood to the retina apparently get narrower before raised blood pressure turns into hypertension; in fact, an ophthalmologist can spot the narrowing before blood pressure goes up at all. An investigation in Sydney, Australia, called the Blue Mountain Eye Study, found that those with narrowed blood vessels in the eyes were twice as likely as those with normal arterioles to develop hypertension over a five-year period. Those predictions of hypertension were independent of other factors including smoking, weight and even blood pressure levels at the start of the study.

The retinas of the 3,654 Sydney residents who participated in the study were photographed with special cameras. Participants were mostly 49 years of age or older. While the changes in the retinal arterioles predicted hypertension regardless of age, the association was strongest for those younger than 65.

This study confirmed the findings of another project, the Atherosclerosis Risk in Communities Study that found that retinal blood vessel narrowing predicted hypertension within three years. Doctors point out that by knowing the risk of future blood pressure problems one can immediately take steps to modify lifestyle to avoid them.

Hypertension is also more prevalent in patients with glaucoma, according to researchers in England who worked with more than 27,000 subjects who had the eye disease.

Doctors in that study speculate that sodium retention may be the underlying cause of both glaucoma and hypertension.

Conversely, controlling blood pressure may be a way to prevent glaucoma. Investigators at the University of Wisconsin found that a reduction in blood pressure was associated with reduced pressure in the eye, known as intraocular pressure. Since intraocular pressure is said to be the most important risk factor for glaucoma, treating blood pressure levels before they reach the hypertension stages may first reduce intraocular pressure and subsequently prevent hypertension and glaucoma.

Fermented milk

People in Scandinavia love fermented milk and enjoy it frequently as a beverage. Fermented milk is sold in several European countries. Good for them, because that fermented milk appears to reduce blood pressure. And good for us since the same bacterium, Lactobacillus, that is present in fermented milk is also found in 'live' yogurt that we can all find in our grocery shops.

How do those bacteria provide their benefits in controlling blood pressure? The Lactobacilli break down the milk protein casein into two types of protein fragments termed tripeptides. (These are isoleucine/praline/praline and valine/praline/praline for those nutritionists and others who might want to know.) Those tripeptides, in turn, block the blood pressure-raising kidney-derived enzyme called angiotensin converting enzyme. You might find that to be a mouthful, but you may well have heard about ACE inhibitors, which are anti-hypertensive prescription drugs. So those milk tripeptides work the same way as the powerful ACE inhibitor drugs.

Finnish researchers worked with 94 participants with hypertension who were not taking anti-hypertensive drugs. They received either 150ml of fermented milk or a non-fermented control drink twice daily for ten weeks. The milk reduced systolic pressure by an average of four points and the diastolic pressure by two points. An insignificant improvement, you scoff? Studies have shown that a three-point reduction in systolic blood pressure cuts stroke risk by 10–13 per cent and the chances of a heart attack by 7 per cent. That's very significant.

If you're a yogurt lover, make sure you look for products whose labels declare 'live' cultures. Enjoyed twice a day, say with breakfast and for a snack, you might be able to get your BP down quite a bit.

Fish oil

We know for certain that those who eat fish, especially cold-water fatty fish such as salmon, herring and sardines, have some protection against cardiovascular disease. But can fish oil supplements provide similar protection? Specifically can those supplements help control blood pressure?

The fish oils that appear to convey heart-health benefits are the omega-3 fatty acids EPA and DHA. Their potential for lowering blood pressure comes through modulating calcium ions inside cells of the body, which signals arterial smooth muscle to dilate, thus narrowing the lumen, the central opening of the artery, and raising blood pressure. The mode of action, then, would be similar to the calcium-channel blocker category of anti-hypertensive drugs.

Studies have, indeed, shown a BP-lowering effect of fish oil supplementation. But doses have been very high, to a point that one would develop 'fish breath' and burping, thus limiting compliance.

Conversely, supplementation with 1,000mg of EPA/DHA (either in purified capsules that concentrate the EPA/DHA or in about 3,000mg of fish oil needed to provide that amount of EPA/DHA) conveys a number of heart-health benefits including reduction of triglyceride levels, improved HDL and lessened blood clotting. That dose would not typically cause the side effects noted above. Would such supplementation improve your blood pressure? It would be worth trying, if you don't already enjoy fish at least two or three days a week, because you'll get those other benefits anyway.

Folic acid

Folic acid is one of the B vitamins. Research has established that consuming about 800 micrograms by way of foods and supplements along with vitamins B6 and B12 reduce levels of the amino acid homocysteine, another risk factor for heart disease. Now recent findings demonstrate that folic acid can also protect against hypertension and the risk of stroke.

In an on-going study with more than 93,000 female nurses, which monitors their lifestyles including diet and physical activity, those who consumed 800 micrograms or more of folic acid daily had a 29 per cent lower risk of high blood pressure than women whose intake was less than 200 micrograms a day. The lead investigator, Dr John Forman, of Boston's Brigham and Women's Hospital, said there is evidence that folic acid has a direct effect on the health of the blood vessel. Most of the women in the study who consumed high levels of folic acid took supplements; it's difficult to get 800 micrograms or more from food alone. That amount would be found in any daily vitamin/mineral supplement plus a B-complex supplement.

Another study, from the Baker Heart Research Institute in Melbourne, Australia, showed that folic acid supplementation for just three weeks reduces both blood pressure in the brachial artery of the arm and arterial stiffness. The investigators concluded that, 'Folic acid is a safe and effective supplement that targets large artery stiffness and may prevent isolated systolic hypertension.'

And researchers in Sweden found that individuals eating a diet rich in green leafy vegetables, beans and other vegetables and fruits had a reduced risk of haemorrhagic stroke. They found a strong connection between levels of folate, the form of the B vitamin found in foods, in the blood and risks of suffering that type of stroke. They did not see a difference in risk in the more common type of stroke termed ischaemic, which is caused by damage or blockage in the arteries providing blood and oxygen to the brain. Perhaps that's because it would be difficult, if not impossible, to reach the protective amount of folic acid, 800 micrograms, noted in the other studies without supplementation.

Garlic

Proving that garlic keeps vampires away would be very difficult, since one would have to find some vampires first in order to do a scientific study. And it appears that proving the benefits of garlic is just as difficult, since one can find data supporting either side of the argument.

The Natural Medicines Comprehensive Database, maintained by the US National Institutes of Health, lists garlic as possibly being effective when taken orally for hypertension. A meta-analysis, combining the data from many trials, showed that garlic decreases systolic BP by an average of 7.7 mmHG and diastolic pressure by 5 mmHG when compared with a placebo. But some placebo-controlled studies have shown no such benefit. And positive studies have been small and uncontrolled. Maybe the differences are due to variations in the formulation or type of garlic powder found in the particular supplement studied.

But most authorities would agree that using fresh, natural garlic cloves in cooking is a healthy thing to do. Fresh garlic cells contain the amino acid alliin, considered to be the most active garlic constituent. When those cells are broken, as when crushing or mincing the cloves, alliin is converted to allicin by the enzyme allinase. It appears that the allicin is effective in the treatment of hypertension by relaxing the smooth muscle in the arteries and so causing vasodilation, the widening of those arteries, allowing freer flow of blood upon demand.

So, if you enjoy garlic in your food, you've got some pretty good justification. It may not keep away vampires, but it could drive some extra health into your heart. Just make sure that the people you're with share that garlic with you or your breath will keep them away as though they were vampires.

Herbs

Many of my readers automatically assume I'm an advocate of herbal remedies because I favour natural approaches to health. Theoretically, the use of herbs makes a lot of sense. They have been used for millennia all over the world. A number of widely prescribed drugs began as botanicals, including aspirin, from willow tree bark, and digitalis, the heart medicine, from the foxglove plant. All well and good. But buying herbs is like buying the proverbial 'pig in a poke'. You have no idea of the purity or concentration of the active ingredients. Other than in Germany, governments provide little or no regulation. You just don't know what you're getting and taking into your body. And that poses the potential for harm as well as benefit.

One study found that 12 out of 14 herbal remedies marketed as treatments for hypertension actually raised blood pressure. Examples include ginkgo, ginseng, liquorice and St John's wort. And other herbs just don't do anything at all. Take the study of hawthorn, a herb used for years, especially in Europe, for the treatment of heart failure and touted as an anti-hypertensive agent. Subjects were divided into one of four groups, and received either hawthorn (500mg of hawthorn leaf extract), magnesium (600mg), a combination of both or a placebo. At the end of a ten-week period there was no difference in blood pressure in any of those four groups. Magnesium, by the way, appears to be effective only when included in an effort to balance *all* electrolytes, including calcium and potassium, to offset the effects of sodium, as explained in Chapter 9.

Laughter

This is one of my personal favourites. To me there's nothing like a good laugh to 'cure what ails you' and there's good research to support the idea that laughter can lower your blood pressure. In fact, the latest data indicate it might be as good for your heart as running or jogging. (But you should really do both.)

How does laughter work? Maybe it counters the ill effects of stress hormones such as adrenaline and cortisol on blood vessel function. Or perhaps it boosts the body's production of nitric oxide, which relaxes the arterial lining and allows for more efficient blood flow. Both modes of action would in turn lower blood pressure. I think it works in a number of ways, those two and others as well.

A study carried out at the University of Maryland Medical Center, in Baltimore, involved healthy men and women whose blood flow through the brachial artery in the arm was measured non-invasively. Doctors use the brachial artery frequently in this sort of research because the dilation of the artery accurately indicates blood flow to and from the heart. Improving arterial dilation helps lower blood pressure.

Measurements were taken before and after the subjects watched either a comedy, *There's Something About Mary*, or a serious, sad film, *Saving Private Ryan*. The researchers found blood vessel dilation to be about 50 per cent better on average after the comedy compared with the serious movie.

I don't own a huge collection of DVDs, but comedies make up a large percentage. No one has yet to quantify laughter with blood pressure control. Do you need to watch a comedy or listen to some good stand-up jokes on a daily basis?

Is one form of humour better than another? To me it doesn't matter. There are some things in life you just know are good for you, and having a good belly laugh regularly is one of them.

Loneliness

Here we come to the flipside of the emotional coin. If laughter has benefit for the heart, one could suppose loneliness would have the opposite effect. Indeed, there is an ever-growing body of evidence that negative energy, whether in the form of anger, hostility or depression, has a nasty effect on heart health. Harvard research linked loneliness in men with higher levels of arterial inflammation than those who were not lonely. A study at Duke University found an increased risk of death from heart disease in isolated individuals. And one of the latest studies links loneliness to high blood pressure.

In those aged over 50 studied at the University of Chicago, the loneliest people had blood pressure readings as much as 30 points higher than those who weren't lonely. The lonelier subjects were, the higher their blood pressure readings. The researchers concluded that loneliness can be as bad for the heart as being overweight or sedentary. And one could well imagine that lonely men and women would also tend to be overweight by way of consolation eating and would be sedentary owing to lack of, perhaps, someone with whom to engage in physical activity.

Earlier research suggests that as many as 11 million Americans aged over 50 often feel isolated, left out or lacking companionship. I would suppose a similar percentage of the British are in the same sad boat.

The next stage of research will be to determine the potential benefit, as measured by blood pressure, of reducing loneliness. But don't wait for the findings to get published. If you feel you're one of the lonely, try your utmost to fill the gap in your life. Don't allow yourself to become mired in self-pity and/or a sense of hopelessness. It's time to make a conscious effort to meet people and make new friends who can provide support and comfort. Build on your own personal likes and loves. Maybe that means volunteering for work through your church. Or joining like-minded bird lovers for walks in the woods. Or enrolling in a sports event such as a ten-pin bowling team. Or reading to children in schools or the elderly in nursing homes. But, please, do something. There's no reason for any of us to be alone. As human beings we are naturally social creatures who need the company of others.

Melatonin

As our bodies' internal clocks determine it's time to sleep, triggered largely by the change from daylight to night darkness, we produce the hormone-like substance melatonin that causes sleepiness. And as melatonin levels in the blood rise, blood pressure levels fall during nightly sleep. Italian researchers speculate that melatonin may decrease noradrenaline levels, increase nitric oxide production, and lessen the resistance to blood flow within large arteries. All those effects would be expected to lower blood pressure.

So the doctors at a clinic in Modena decided to evaluate the effect of melatonin on the daily blood pressure variance in nine women with normal blood pressure and another nine whose hypertension was being treated with ACE inhibitor drugs. Ages ranged from 47 to 63. For three weeks, the women were randomly assigned to slow-release melatonin (1mg released rapidly and 2mg slowly) or a placebo. During the next three weeks, the groups were switched. Those who had been taking a placebo now received melatonin and vice versa.

Melatonin treatment decreased both systolic and diastolic nightly blood pressure by 3.77 and 3.63 points on average. Some women had as much as a 10-point blood pressure decline during the night's sleep. Those who normally had the least reduction in nocturnal BP showed the greatest improvement.

There was no change in blood pressure during the day, which was to be expected since melatonin levels disappear or diminish after waking. But the difference between nocturnal and diurnal BP intensified, and that difference has been linked with heart disease. The larger the difference between BP during the day and during the night the better.

Similar research has been conducted at Harvard University, where investigators gave melatonin to 16 men over a three-week period. A single dose of 2.5mg of melatonin did no good. But taken nightly over the course of the three weeks, it reduced systolic and diastolic BP on average by 6 and 4 points, respectively. The difference between BP during the day and during the night was increased by 15 per cent systolic and 25 per cent diastolic. Subjects enjoyed better sleep as well, though improvement in sleep was not correlated with that of blood pressure.

When I read the first research reports in this area in 2004, I immediately began taking a melatonin tablet every night at bedtime. Why bother if one can't tell any difference since there's no improvement in BP readings during the day? Just as there are typically no symptoms of hypertension, we know it does damage to the arteries and places us at risk of heart attack and stroke. And while we can't 'feel' the increased difference between BP at night and BP during the day, our cardiovascular health will reflect the benefit. Melatonin is very inexpensive. Why not seek that benefit?

The best product would be a controlled-release melatonin that would keep levels of the substance more constant throughout the hours of sleep. One such choice would be Health Yourself C-R Melatonin. But any time-release, sustained-release or controlled-release melatonin would be fine.

Music

Listening to fast tempo music tends to increase blood pressure, while slower music may be useful for lowering BP. Random pauses in a piece of music enhance the pressure-lowering effect.

In a collaborative study, researchers from Italy and the UK played Indian raga, slow classical, fast classical, rap and modern techno music for 12 classically trained musicians and 12 individuals with no musical training. Faster tempo music with simple rhythm patterns increased breathing rate, heart rate and both systolic and diastolic BP. Slower music had less effect and raga significantly lowered heart rate. During two-minute pauses in the music, heart rate, blood pressure and breathing rate decreased even more significantly in both trained and untrained individuals.

This trial appears to contradict other research showing that relaxing, 'meditative' music that is continuous, without pauses, lowers BP. The researchers speculate that all music has pauses, and that concentrating on the music and then lapsing into pauses may have more of a meditative effect.

Over-the-counter (OTC) medication and prescription-only medication (POM)

• Remedies for allergies and colds and occasional flu may play a role in raising your blood pressure that you're not aware of but definitely should be. A meta-analysis of 24 placebo-controlled studies involving a total of 1,285 subjects showed a slight blood-pressure-raising effect of pseudoephedrine, a frequently used decongestant used on its own or in combination with antihistamines. The effect might be greatest in older individuals and those whose BP is already higher than it should be.

- Painkillers and anti-inflammatory agents may also pose a problem. Watch out for paracetamol (Panadol – OTC), naproxen (Naprosyn – POM only) and ibuprofen (Advil, Motrin – both OTC).
- Weight loss products frequently contain stimulants including bitter orange (*Citrus aurantium*), caffeine, ma huang and gaurana. These are meant to depress appetite and to increase energy, thus burning more calories. Often these substances are used in combination, such as caffeine and bitter orange. That particular combination may increase heart rate and blood pressure and create a risk for adverse cardiovascular events, especially for those with existing conditions. Consumerlab.com research has determined that products can contain as much caffeine as six cans of cola, in one case, and 14 cans in another. All such stimulants, especially in high doses, have BP-raising potential.
- Most younger men and women don't think of 'energy drinks' as drugs, but they contain the same stimulants as weight loss products and have the same potential for raising both heart rate and blood pressure. They also pose a risk of dehydration, especially when used at parties and clubs when dancing. I agree with many health authorities who believe those energy drinks are a disaster waiting to happen, particularly when used to excess.
- Doctors at the Mayo Clinic, in Rochester, Minnesota, warn that, 'If you have high blood pressure and it's not responding to treatment, it could be because of a medication you're taking.' Whether you use the non-drug approaches detailed in this book or take prescription anti-hypertensive drugs or both, be aware that a number of other

prescribed drugs can cancel out their BP-lowering potential. Such prescription drugs include anti-depressants such as bupropion (Zyban), anti-inflammatory agents including celecoxib (Celebrex) and oral contraceptives. Women over 35 or who are overweight or drink alcohol to excess are at most risk of developing high blood pressure while taking the pill, but any woman may be affected. Fortunately, most hormonal contraceptives today contain only low-level doses of oestrogen or progesterone or both. Those with more than 50 micrograms of oestrogen are most likely to raise blood pressure.

Other drugs that may cause or worsen hypertension include most non-steroidal anti-inflammatory drugs, corticosteroids, liquorice, immunosuppressive drugs, as might be taken to prevent rejection of an organ transplant or manage HIV infection, various cough medicines, appetite suppressants, decongestants, eye drops and amphetamines.

Sleep disorders

We all know how a good night's sleep can make the next day more productive and enjoyable. Doctors also know the importance of sleep and how sleep deprivation, common in today's hectic lifestyle, can have a negative impact on health in a number of ways. Perhaps, in fact, your sleep habits are influencing your blood pressure.

Research from Columbia University, in New York, links insufficient sleep with raised blood pressure. In that study, investigators found that sleeping less than six hours a night more than doubled the risk of developing hypertension. That remained true even after factoring in variables such as obesity and diabetes. Subjects ranged in age from 32 to 59.

Why might getting less than recommended amounts of sleep predispose a person to high blood pressure? Pressure levels are lower during sleep than during waking hours. The difference between night and day pressures protects against hypertension; the greater the difference, subtracting one from the other, the greater the protection. Thus sleeping fewer than the recommended eight hours nightly would expose one to daytime blood pressures for a longer period of time, and the longer that sleep deprivation, the higher average pressures will be.

A condition termed sleep apnoea may be even more deadly. Those who suffer with this disorder have difficulty breathing during sleep. Sleep studies have shown patients waking as often as once a minute. This keeps them from ever slipping into a solid, restful sleep. Such individuals actually stop breathing and then abruptly awaken and resume breathing. Snoring, often extremely loud and disturbing to partners, is common.

Scientists believe there is a causal link between sleep apnoea and hypertension. Alleviating the disorder by surgically removing tissue that blocks the airway or by pumping air into the nostrils by way of a machine can lower blood pressure. Those suffering from sleep apnoea are often obese.

This extreme form of sleep disturbance has also been implicated in causing strokes. Snoring is no laughing matter.

If you suffer from any form of sleep disorder, discuss this fully with your doctor as part of your blood pressure management.

Vitamin supplements

While there's no question that a diet rich in fruits and vegetables and whole grains can very effectively lower blood pressure, the same can't be said for vitamin supplements. At the least, clinical trials have come up with mixed results and aren't very encouraging.

Vitamin E appears to have no effect on blood pressure. A randomised, controlled, though open-label (not double-blind, see page 232) trial measured blood pressure in 142 patients with controlled hypertension. There was no change with vitamin E in systolic BP and a small reduction of 1.6 points diastolic.

Vitamin C appears to be more promising. Theoretically this vitamin functions as an antioxidant that would enhance the synthesis or prevent the breakdown of nitric oxide, a naturally occurring gas produced in the lining of the arteries that keeps those vessels flexible and more capable of vasodilation. Studies have shown reductions in systolic BP though not in diastolic pressure when subjects were treated with vitamin C. A randomised, placebo-controlled trial with 39 patients yielded interesting results. Subjects took a 2g 'loading dose' and then 500mg daily for 30 days. Systolic BP was reduced by 13mmHg, but diastolic pressure was not affected.

Other trials were not as positive. Moreover, millions of men and women who routinely take at least 500mg of vitamin C daily, and who have done so for many years, develop hypertension. Supplementation with vitamins C and E may have other benefits, and I think they probably do, but I wouldn't count on either to bring BP down.

Chapter 14

Secret Weapons Against the Silent Killer

More than two decades ago I began my search for ways to lower my own cholesterol levels and avoid an early death from heart disease. Certainly the essential foundation of such a programme had to include increased physical activity and a heart-healthy diet. But knowing that other factors entered into the cholesterol picture – notably that the body makes 80 per cent of all the cholesterol in the bloodstream – I realised that I needed something more than diet and exercise. My search led me to the soluble fibres in oat bran and other foods that actually 'flush' out cholesterol, and the vitamin niacin to stop the body's excessive production. Since that time, I've found additional, natural approaches to lowering cholesterol, including plant sterols, known as phytosterols, red yeast rice, pantethine, and policosanol.

And so it was with a sense of déjà vu that I began my own search for ways to normalise blood pressure. I've detailed the foundation of a solid programme in the chapters of this book, and those lifestyle elements are, again, essential. But by the time most people recognise the importance of blood pressure in heart health, their blood pressure has already begun to creep up. Thus it's not just a matter of prevention, but one of a vital need for a 'cure', for a way to get blood pressure down safely and effectively. My research has been thrilling for me. And the results I've achieved are as dramatic as those I managed for cholesterol. And so it's with a great deal of delight that I guide you through what I've learned about the 'Secret Weapons' against high blood pressure.

You're about to read a wonderful story that took decades to develop by way of research all over the world. It's a medical detective tale, complete with mystery and discovery. Three of the major characters won the Nobel Prize in medicine. Four plant-derived supplements are recognised for their abilities to lower blood pressure naturally. And thanks to all those efforts, you and I are the real winners in our fight against hypertension.

When we talk about heart disease, we're really talking about a disease of the arteries that supply blood to the heart muscle, known as the coronary arteries. A heart attack occurs when the coronary arteries cannot get enough blood to the heart muscle, because of a blockage, and it begins to die from lack of oxygen. Similarly, a stroke happens when the carotid arteries in the neck can't provide sufficient blood and oxygen to the brain, most typically when a clot forms in a narrowed carotid artery. In any discussion about cholesterol, smoking, blood pressure and other risk factors, what tends to be forgotten is the importance of those arteries themselves.

When most people think about the arteries at all, it's in terms of plumbing. The arteries are simply pipes, conduits, for blood flow. Problems occur when those pipes get clogged, though not in the simplistic way commonly imagined. The plaque, as arterial blockage is properly termed, doesn't accumulate on the inner wall of the artery the way calcium builds up in bathroom pipes. Rather, it's a complex process that develops inside the layers of the wall of that artery.

How and why does that blockage occur? For many years, the vast majority of researchers focused on the blockage itself, disregarding the 'pipe' that was being clogged. Studies beginning in the 1950s showed a correlation between cholesterol levels and cardiovascular disease. Other risk factors including cigarette smoking and hypertension were also revealed. Then we learned that the principal 'villain' in the cholesterol family is LDL, and that HDL is the 'good guy'. LDL circulates in the bloodstream and forms an arterial blockage when levels become excessive. HDL does exactly the opposite, carrying cholesterol away from the tissues and back to the liver, where it can be disposed of.

Painstaking investigations gradually described the chemical and cellular processes by which LDL penetrates the lining of the artery and, in concert with a variety of blood cells and smooth muscle cells and other materials, slowly but surely builds up clumps of plaque in the walls of the artery. It was quite logical to seek ways that those processes could be interrupted to prevent or slow the blockage that would limit blood flow and that could result in heart attack or stroke.

Healthy arteries, healthy heart and circulation

Certainly we still want to keep levels of LDL, triglycerides, glucose and blood pressure at optimum levels. We know that by doing so we can slow, stop and even reverse the disease process. But there's another way of looking at heart disease. Instead of looking at the blockage itself, and the materials that form that blockage, scientists today are concentrating more and more on the artery.

At this point in the story, I must introduce some terms that you're probably not familiar with and that you may never have heard of. It's like learning the strange, unpronounceable names of characters in a fantasy book such as *Lord of the Rings*.

Let's start by saying that the artery wall is not a solid tube like a bathroom pipe. Rather, there are three layers, as shown in the illustration below: the inner layer is called the *intima*, the middle layer is the *media*, and the outer layer is the *adventitia*. Finally, separating the muscle layers of the artery from the flow of blood through the central open space, or *lumen*, there is a lining of flat cells called the *endothelium*.

In the past, doctors used the term 'hardening of the arteries'. While we don't hear that expression used much any more, it's still an important concept. The medical term for this is *arteriosclerosis*, from the Greek words for artery and hardening or stiffening. Heart disease is now known to be much more complicated than simply hardening of the arteries and so the word most commonly used to describe it is *atherosclerosis*, combining the Greek words for 'gruel' and hardening. Atherosclerosis describes heart disease very well, since the disease is characterised by hardening of the artery *and* a deposition of plaque that has the consistency of gruel or porridge in the arterial walls.

Think about that for a moment. When we're young, our arteries are nice and flexible, without any blockage. As we age, the arteries stiffen and become blocked by plaque deposits, both of which limit the flow of blood. Kids can play games and sports that get the heart beating like crazy, forcing blood through soft, elastic arteries to the muscles that need more oxygen, all without risk. But if adults overexert themselves or experience extreme stress, the blocked and hardened arteries can't get blood through to the muscles of the heart or to the brain. Sometimes a plaque ruptures, spilling out its contents into the bloodstream where a clot forms. Small clots can travel through even narrowed arteries. But large clots can get stuck, stopping the blood flow. The result is a heart attack or stroke.

Here's how we tie these, perhaps seemingly unrelated, concepts together. Over the course of a lifetime, the endothelium lining of the artery is subjected to a series of tiny injuries. Innocently enough, the body tries to heal itself, to repair those little rips in the endothelium. It does so by bringing in blood cells, LDL and muscle cells to form a kind of 'seal'. Over a period of time that 'seal' grows larger and larger and the plaque inside the walls of the artery bulges outwards into the lumen, slowing the flow of blood. At the same time, as we age, our arteries stiffen and are no longer capable of stretching like rubber bands to expand and allow extra blood flow when needed. Blood pressure gradually increases, sometimes to the point of hypertension.

Recognising that both the arterial plaque and the artery itself are involved in the disease process, scientists today approach the problem from both directions. But the research effort is slow, spanning the course of decades. Imagine a huge jigsaw puzzle, put together one piece at a time until the final picture emerges. Sometimes scientists believe they 'see' the picture, only to find out years later that a missing piece of the puzzle now reveals a very different picture. The good news is that we have put more of those pieces of the puzzle together and we're getting a clearer view of the picture of cardio-vascular disease than we've ever had before.

The smoking gun

Researchers stumbled upon one piece of the puzzle in the picture of a healthy endothelium in the late 1980s. They realised that the endothelium itself released some sort of substance that promoted 'compliance', the medical word for elasticity and flexibility, of the artery. Whatever 'it' was, 'it' was released, performed its action, and disappeared in a fraction of a second. Trying to identify that mysterious substance was like grabbing a handful of smoke. But even before identifying it, investigators began to study the manner in which 'it' kept the artery healthy. Rather than referring to it as 'it' they came up with the term EDRF, standing for endothelium-derived relaxation factor.

For years, articles in the medical literature detailed the activities and functions of EDRF. Even before they knew what it was, scientists recognised the enormous importance of

EDRF. Despite the difficulty of isolating and identifying something that appeared and disappeared in a nanosecond, EDRF was discovered to be a gas, nitric oxide (NO). That discovery earned three doctors the Nobel Prize in medicine in 1998.

Although EDRF/NO is relatively new in the world of pharmacology, its impact has been enormous. In just 25 years more than 31,000 papers have been published with NO in the title and more than 65,000 refer to it in some way. That represents a lot of work, pieces of the jigsaw puzzle put together in laboratories, clinics and medical centres globally!

After identification, the next step was to determine how NO was made in the endothelium. As with other bodily substances, NO manufacture involves a pathway that requires other chemical entities. The substrate or 'raw material' required is an amino acid, a building block of protein, called l-arginine, and henceforth in this book referred to simply as arginine. A special enzyme, endothelial nitric oxide synthase (eNOS), must be present for NO to be made from arginine. Both of those discoveries were made in 1993. A year earlier a different form of arginine, asymmetrical dimethyl arginine (ADMA), was found to inhibit NO synthesis.

Blood pressure is strongly influenced by the amount of NO in the blood. In addition to relaxing the arteries and making them more compliant and able to constrict and dilate as needed, NO inhibits what doctors refer to as ACE, angiotensin-I converting enzyme, which raises blood pressure. Indeed, one of the commonly prescribed anti-hypertensive category of drugs is that of the ACE inhibitors. As we age, levels of NO decline and, not surprisingly, blood pressure goes up. It should be apparent to the most casual observer that if we can increase NO production, arteries will get healthier, ACE will be inhibited and blood pressure will go down. This is the mode of action, the 'war plan', of the 'Secret Weapons' against blood pressure.

If NO could be bottled as tablets or capsules, it would be declared a wonder drug and would make a pharmaceutical company a huge fortune. This simple little gas comprised of one molecule of nitrogen and one of oxygen performs a variety of wonders in the body. For example, NO

- improves the ability of arteries to dilate,
- inhibits blood cells called platelets from aggregating and forming clots,
- limits production of smooth muscle cells that contribute to formation of arterial plaque,
- regulates the oxygenation of cells,
- mediates cellular defence systems, and
- functions as a neurotransmitter in both the central and peripheral nervous systems.

As we age, the body produces less and less NO, especially when LDL cholesterol levels are high, when we smoke cigarettes, when we gain weight, when we live a sedentary lifestyle, and when we develop type 2 diabetes and sugar levels rise in the blood. Reduced production of NO leads to arterial constriction that limits blood flow, raises blood pressure and increases blood clot production, leading to more rapid cell death and cardiovascular disease. For reasons yet to be determined, Afro-Caribbean people produce less NO than white people, which may explain why the incidence of hypertension is higher in those communities. And while there is an association, we don't know whether decreased production of NO contributes to the development of type 2 diabetes or whether that form of diabetes results in less NO. Decreased NO production has also been correlated with early development of atherosclerosis. At the Scientific Sessions of the American Heart Association, in 2005, Russian scientists reported their findings that a decline in NO production parallels increases in blood pressure from mild to severe.

You don't need a doctorate in scientific research or a medical degree to see why it would be nice if our bodies produced more NO. But it did take hundreds of men and women with those qualifications and others, working in labs and medical centres internationally, to work out some ways to maintain and increase NO production. You and I owe those people a huge debt, and following the recommendations stemming from their findings will help us to lower our blood pressure and reduce our risk of heart attack and stroke.

As noted earlier, known risk factors for heart disease and hypertension in general, including high LDL counts, smoking, obesity and sedentary behaviour, contribute to decreased production of NO in the endothelium. So we have more reason to get those factors under control.

I spoke of pharmaceutical companies earlier. It's no surprise that the pharmaceutical industry is hard at work developing drugs to improve NO status. One now being introduced is nebivolol (Nebilet), a drug in the beta-blocker family frequently prescribed by doctors to treat hypertension. Nebivolol is said to increase NO in the endothelium more than other beta-blockers. But all have side effects, as detailed in Chapter 15.

It would be better if we could boost NO production without drugs. We can do just that with four unique antioxidants taken as dietary supplements. So now we turn to the pay-off in this story, with four ways to increase NO and protect our arteries while lowering blood pressure dramatically.

Weapon number one - arginine

Let's start with this one because arginine is the raw material, the substrate, from which NO is made in the endothelium. To get the job done, one must have an adequate amount of eNOS (endothelial nitric oxide synthase), the enzyme that acts as a catalyst in the production process, and enough of the amino acid arginine. But the process can be blocked by high levels of ADMA (asymmetric dimethylarginine), a known inhibitor of NO synthesis.

What can we do to help in the process? At this time, testing for ADMA is rare, restricted to major research centres. That's a shame, since high ADMA levels have been associated with nearly quadrupling the risk of heart attack and stroke by undermining the health of the endothelium, a condition known as endothelial dysfunction. But, on a practical level, you won't have access to ADMA testing. That said, one can override ADMA by increasing blood concentrations of arginine. Sufficient arginine, in turn, leads to production of adequate amounts of eNOS. And with enough arginine and eNOS present in the arteries, the endothelium can produce NO. We can optimise NO, and lessen endothelial dysfunction, then, by supplementing with arginine. Numerous studies have demonstrated the benefits of arginine supplementation. In 12 studies from 1991 to 2005, arginine was shown to improve blood flow by improving endothelial function. Seven out of ten people showed significant reduction in angina pain, which results from insufficient blood and oxygen reaching the heart muscle, the myocardium. Another investigation showed the benefits of arginine in improving exercise capacity. Patients suffering from congestive heart failure showed a significant improvement in blood flow, arterial compliance (elasticity and flexibility to allow for greater dilation) and heart function.

Men, in particular, will appreciate another benefit of arginine and subsequent increase of NO. Cardiovascular disease affects not only the arteries supplying blood to the heart muscle and brain but also the arteries channelling blood into the penis to achieve an erection. As those penile arteries harden and become blocked with atherosclerotic plaques, the resulting reduced blood flow leads to what is now termed erectile dysfunction (ED), the medical term for male impotence. Viagra (sildenafil) is one drug in a family of agents that improves erectile dysfunction; they all share the same mode of action: increasing production of NO to improve arterial blood flow. In fact, Viagra was first investigated as a drug for heart patients – ED improvement was a fortuitous 'side effect'. Taking oral arginine supplements has been shown to have the same benefit.

Pulmonary hypertension is a very different disease from the more common systemic hypertension. It occurs in patients with sickle-cell disease and sometimes in the newborn. Pulmonary hypertension, it now appears, involves arginine metabolism and NO availability. Arginine supplements have been shown to improve this disease by increasing levels of substrate for NO production.

I have been following the research into arginine and NO for many years. But there has been a major stumbling block limiting the practicality of supplementing with arginine. The studies I've referred to thus far have used either intravenous administration of arginine to achieve high concentrations in the endothelium in a short period of time or extremely large oral doses of arginine supplements. How large? Doctors have given patients doses from 5g to 15g daily, with most studies averaging 8–9g.

Typical arginine supplements provide 500mg of the amino acid per capsule. That's half a gram. To get, for example, 9g of arginine, one would have to swallow 18 capsules a day, on an hourly basis for best effect. That would be both impractical and very expensive. Oral arginine is absorbed and metabolised rapidly. The majority of a given dose would be gone in less than an hour.

In reading and hearing about the work with arginine in clinical settings, and the drawbacks of arginine supplements, I was reminded of my experiences with niacin, used to lower levels of LDL cholesterol and raise HDL counts. There was no doubt, going back literally decades, that niacin was wonderfully effective. But it was seldom recommended by doctors because research in the 1970s and into the 1980s indicated the need for very high doses, which far too frequently resulted in what were termed 'nuisance' side effects of flushing and gastric upset. While doctors might consider those mere nuisances, patients simply refused to take niacin. Then, in the late 1980s, about the time my cholesterol book was published, a small company developed a sustained-release formulation that drastically reduced both the dose and side effects of niacin. I go into detail on that product, Endur-acin, on page 165. Could there be a sustained-release arginine?

In 2004, Thorne Research developed the first such product, which they call Perfusia-SR. Each capsule contains 350mg, with directions to take three capsules twice daily – morning and evening. Dr Alan L. Miller, technical adviser at Thorne, advises patients to take the capsules in the morning with breakfast and at dinner in the evening. That adds up to just over 2g, far short of the 8–9g previously used. But thanks to the sustained-release formulation, arginine remains in the blood for the entire day and night, working its wonders. Thus it's not necessary to consume those large doses.

Research done at the University of Texas by Dr Lance Gould provided dramatic evidence of arginine's potential. Dr Gould is a recognised expert in cardiac imaging, taking pictures of the heart at work. He used a technique called a PET scan; that stands for positron emission tomography. PET scans show how well the heart is being 'perfused', supplied with blood through the coronary arteries, and does so in colours reflecting the heart muscle getting less or more blood and oxygen. He took PET images before and after patients received Perfusia-SR. You can see the results for yourself by visiting the website www.thorne.com. Sustained-release arginine taken over one month greatly increased blood and oxygen perfusion of the heart.

Of the 29 volunteers in the study, 63 per cent experienced a drop in blood pressure as well. Systolic blood pressure came down by an average of 4.1 mmHG and diastolic was reduced by an average of 3.7 mmHG. But those are averages across the board, whether or not the subjects had raised blood pressure to begin with. Individuals with normal blood pressure, or just slightly raised, showed little or no benefit. But those who were borderline or hypertensive (more than 130/85 mmHG) achieved a systolic reduction averaging 10.5 mmHG with a diastolic drop of 4.9 mmHG. Those improvements are comparable to ones achieved with prescription drugs. I expect – and hope – that we'll see much more research with sustained-release arginine in the future. This is a new frontier.

I've asked a number of doctors in private practice – 'real world' doctors, not those in university research centres – to experiment a bit with newly diagnosed blood pressure patients. The results have been terrific. One doctor, a family doctor in Florida, was so amazed that he telephoned with something close to disbelief in his voice. The patient was a 40-year-old male with a blood pressure of 155/102 mmHG on average. After taking Perfusia-SR for one month, that pressure was down to 120/73 mmHG. It appears that the higher the blood pressure to begin with, the better the results will be.

But here's the sad story behind the reason why I selected that particular patient to tell you about. After hearing the results, I said to Dr Walsh in Florida, 'Of course you gave him the information for reordering the arginine so he can maintain those good results.' Sadly, that was not the case. It turned out that it was less expensive for the man to get a prescription drug through his insurance plan than for him to buy the side-effect-free supplement, and the patient elected to take the drug. The moral of this little story is that ultimately it will be your decision to do nothing and remain at risk, pay for a harmless and very helpful dietary supplement or take a prescription drug.

I must, however, disclose one study that showed a risk in taking arginine supplements. Researchers at Johns Hopkins Medical Center, in Baltimore, Maryland, worked with 153 patients who had had a heart attack just three to 21 days before being given either 9g – 3g three times daily – of arginine or a placebo, for six months. Of those patients, 77 were over 60 years of age. During that period, there were 12 cardiovascular events (heart attack, death and hospitalisation for heart failure) in the arginine group and seven in the placebo group. There were six deaths in the arginine group and none in the placebo group.

How could that have happened? Well, one must look beyond the newspaper headlines. The subjects were seriously ill following those heart attacks. One died from a rupture in the heart muscle; this would certainly not be associated with arginine in any way. Two died from sepsis, severe infections. Certainly this is going to stimulate additional research. But in the meantime I don't feel that one isolated study should negate the positive findings of all other studies. I am reminded of a lone journal article that got a lot of attention in its day back in the 1990s reporting that there was no cholesterol improvement in those taking phytosterols, the plant sterols now known to lower levels by 10 per cent on average. That article still makes researchers scratch their collective heads but prior and subsequent findings put it in the category of fluke. I think the same will be true for this l-arginine study. Personally, I still take the sustained-release l-arginine.

In addition to its blood-pressure-lowering benefits, arginine, especially in the sustained-release formulation that keeps a more or less constant level in the bloodstream, promotes the health of the endothelium. That's been well established in a large number of clinical studies. Remember that arginine is the body's *only* substrate, or raw material, for NO production. Without sufficient supplies in the body, we cannot make enough NO for optimal arterial health.

For reasons not totally understood yet – and I'm certain that as time goes on, we'll have more and more knowledge, owing to the incredible importance of this new field of heart health – arginine works best for those with a blood pressure of more than 130/80 mmHG. Those in the lower categories, termed pre-hypertension, inexplicably could take arginine without seeing any improvement, while those with much higher numbers, such as Dr Walsh's patient, will experience a complete normalisation.

For more information on Perfusia-SR, visit the websites www.perfusia.com (for sales information) and www.thorne.com (for additional research details including before and after PET scan images).

While Thorne was the first company to develop a sustained-release arginine capsule, a company with an outstanding performance record and an international reputation in sustained-release formulations has perfected a 350mg tablet that delivers even more predictable and consistent blood levels of arginine. The Endurance Products Company, of Tigard, Oregon, now markets this product as EP L-Arginine SR. Having developed a unique system of sustained-release delivery of other supplements including, for example, niacin and vitamin C, Endurance Products arginine can be completely trusted to provide maximum benefit. Their system of sustained release of arginine is actually superior. Another major difference is a significantly lower price for the product itself as well as for shipping. Delivery outside the US is handled by Pharmaceutical Trade Services, Inc. You can place orders by e-mail at www.endur.com; click on Customer Services, International Orders.

I hereby disclose that I have absolutely no financial interest in any of the products or companies I have discussed in this chapter. I receive no compensation of any kind from purchase of any or all of the 'Special Weapons'.

The good news is that there are more weapons in our blood-pressure-lowering armoury. And the next one we'll consider has been shown to do a wonderful job of dealing with those lower levels of raised blood pressure.

Weapon number two – grape seed extract

Grapes have been held in high regard for promoting health since ancient times. One can find references to recommendations for increased grape eating by doctors, including Hippocrates, virtually everywhere in the world where grapes have been grown. Grapes and their vines decorate everything from clothing and vases throughout history. Dr John Harvey Kellogg, the man who began the Kellogg cereal empire, prescribed 10–14lb (yes, pounds, not grams or even ounces) of grapes daily as a remedy for high blood pressure. No, don't worry, I'm not going to suggest that you do that! Fortunately we've learned a lot since those days, and the solution is a lot more practical.

While you may never have heard of Dr Kellogg's grape obsession, you certainly know about what's called the 'French paradox'. Why does France have a remarkably low rate of death from heart disease despite a diet rich in the foods most health authorities tell us to cut back on? Could it be the red wine that the French wash those foods down with?

Actually, subsequent studies – and there have been hundreds of them – have determined that the major benefit of regular wine consumption comes from the alcohol, which raises levels of the protective HDL cholesterol (see page 148). Along those lines, beer, spirits, other wines or whatever might be your drink of choice will do the same thing. But there is something very special about red wine, which gets its colour from having the grape skins left in the vats during the fermentation process. White wine lacks the red colour because the skins are removed. We've learned that the red colour comes from a special class of plant substances called polyphenols, powerful agents that came under scientific scrutiny only in the mid-1900s. There are literally thousands of polyphenols in fruits, vegetables and all plants and plant-derived foods. Why did it take science so long to recognise the value of these substances? Probably the biggest reason research got a slow start was and still is the enormous diversity and complexity of their chemical structures.

Relax, there's no reason for you to learn the intricate nuances of the wonderful world of polyphenols. Suffice to say that current data support very strongly a combination of polyphenols in their roles in prevention and/or cure of cardiovascular diseases, cancers, diabetes and degenerative nerve diseases. Although polyphenols have been under the scientific microscope for just over a decade, the wealth of knowledge built up thus far is fantastic, and new information is being added to the scientific and medical literature in journals all over the world every week. In fact, the internationally renowned *American Journal of Clinical Nutrition* devoted an entire 120-page, 17-article supplement to 'Dietary Polyphenols and Health' along with its January 2005 issue.

Much of the polyphenol research has concentrated on cardiovascular disease, and today it is well established that polyphenols, consumed as foods or supplements, improve health status and reduce cardiovascular risk. Much of that body of investigation has involved laboratory animals, but we now have enough human clinical studies to prove their benefits for us as well as for mice and rats. One such study showed how rats given grape seed extract following induced heart attacks had far less damage. In fact, my own interest in grape seed extract, a particularly rich source of particular poly-phenols, began in 2003 when I read that when it was fed to mice their blood pressures came down appreciably. I wrote about that study in my newsletter, and began adding grape seed extract to my own supplement regimen. To my delight, I saw a very nice improvement. But more about blood pressure control in just a bit.

Any reading about polyphenols in the medical journals inevitably leads us back to the health of the endothelium and the role of nitric oxide (NO). Truly, that's where the action is, with good reason, since NO has vital abilities to help arterial dilation, prevent inflammation, limit formation of blood clots and, in general, promote arterial health. And in that special *AJCN* supplement, one of the most prominently discussed sources of polyphenols was grape seed extract (GSE). That's because GSE has one of the highest concentrations of those potent substances. Just a little bit goes a long way.

To get the natural antioxidant and artery-protecting benefits of just one 200mg grape seed extract tablet or capsule, one would have to drink 100ml of red wine, 175ml of red grape juice or a serving of various fruits. To think that for centuries grape seeds were discarded as waste during the production of wine!

When postmenopausal women took a daily dose of 100–500mg of grape seed extract, they lowered their systolic pressure by 20 points. Interestingly, the salt content in the diet of those women was particularly high. A better recommendation, I would think, would be to ease up on the salt while taking grape seed extract tablets or capsules.

Much of the investigation into the benefits of GSE has been carried out at the University of California at Davis by the professor of cardiovascular medicine, C. Tissa Kappagoda. At the Experimental Biology Conference in San Diego, in April 2003, he and his associates presented the findings of three such studies. Dr Kappagoda described GSE as 'a powerful antioxidant' that has a significant effect on atherosclerosis by preventing cholesterol from accumulating in the arteries.

In two of the studies, the UC Davis team gave GSE along with a high-fat diet to guinea pigs. After 12 weeks, the cholesterol accumulation in the animals' arteries was significantly lower in the group receiving GSE. A third study they described at that meeting showed that GSE inhibited the atherosclerotic effects of the highly saturated fat in coconut oil.

But you and I are neither rats, nor mice, nor guinea pigs. The good news is that research has shown benefits for humans as well. One study showed how GSE 'supercharged' vitamins E and C in humans to provide greater antioxidant capabilities than the vitamins alone. A British project revealed how the polyphenols of GSE help to restore endothelial function by inhibiting a substance called endothelin-1. But most recently have come truly exciting breakthroughs in the use of GSE to lower blood pressure in two types of patients.

The first investigation, also done by the UC Davis team, involved 24 male and female patients diagnosed with what is termed 'metabolic syndrome', categorised by overweight, insulin resistance and resultant higher levels of blood glucose, low counts of protective HDL cholesterol along with high concentrations of triglycerides and raised blood pressure. The patients were divided into three groups of eight. The first received a placebo, the second was given 150mg of a specially formulated GSE, and the third took 300mg of GSE. For one month, participants' blood pressure readings were auto-matically measured and recorded every 12 hours.

While there was no blood pressure change in the placebo group, Dr Kappagoda first announced at the 26 March 2006 meeting of the American Chemical Society that participants in the other two groups achieved an equal degree of BP reduction, averaging 12 mmHG systolic and 8 mmHG diastolic. Those taking the 300mg dose also reduced their serum LDL cholesterol. The higher the LDL to begin with, the better the improvement.

Dr Kappagoda conducted a second investigation of the remarkable capabilities of MegaNatural BP, this time with men and women diagnosed with pre-hypertension, with systolic levels of from 120 to 139 and diastolic BP of 80 to 89. Pre-hypertension is estimated to affect 31 per cent of the entire US population, 39 per cent of men and 23 per cent of women. Counter to popular belief, those elevated blood pressure levels now termed pre-hypertension affect more than 37 per cent of African-Americans, 32.2 per cent of whites, and 30.9 per cent of Hispanics between 20 and 39 years of age – not just middle-aged and older persons.

Subjects in the UC Davis pre-hypertension study had a baseline systolic pressure averaging 134.1 and a diastolic reading of 79.1 Thirty participants completed the study. As Dr Kappagoda reported in April at the 2007 meeting of the Federation of American Societies for Experimental Biology, blood pressures were measured automatically at the start, midpoint and end of the eight-week study. Again, no difference was noted in the blood pressures of the placebo group. But those in the group receiving 300 mg of MegaNatural BP daily had average reductions down to 125.8 systolic and 73.4 diastolic. That means a lowering of about 8 points systolic and 6 points diastolic. Such reductions can significantly reduce the risk of heart attack and stroke.

While grape seed extract has been shown to have a blood-pressure-lowering effect in the past in other studies, it was pleasantly surprising to see such impressive improvements with rather low GSE doses. Based on previous animal studies, which usually correlate pretty closely on a milligram-dose-per-kilogram-weight basis to humans, one would have predicted the need for much higher doses to achieve that sort of BP lowering.

The reason is a specially formulated grape seed extract that concentrates the isolate found to be the responsible entity that lowers blood pressure. It is made by the Polyphenolics company and sold as MegaNatural BP grape seed extract under a variety of brands as well as directly from the company. While one might expect BP lowering from ordinary GSE, no detailed human studies have been carried out to establish necessary doses, though they would be significantly higher than those needed with the MegaNatural BP.

Visit the website www.polyphenolics.com to obtain MegaNatural BP grape seed extract. Unfortunately ordinary formulations of grape seed extract will not provide blood-pressure-lowering effects.

What about drinking grape juice? It's a wonderful source of polyphenols, and I strongly recommend it. You'll find a number of ways of using grape juice concentrate in the recipe section at the end of the book. But to get a major benefit, you'd have to drink a lot of grape juice every day. In another study reported at the 2003 meeting of the Federation of American Societies for Experimental Biology, men who drank 350ml of red grape juice daily for 12 weeks saw a drop in systolic blood pressure from 142.7 to 137.0 mmHG while diastolic pressure went down from 87.9 to 82.1 mmHG. That's nice, but I wonder how practical it would be in real life.

Weapon number three – tomato extract

Even those who have been taking BP-lowering drugs will benefit from this natural choice. And those who are determined to get that BP down without drugs will benefit enormously. Tomato extract, which is rich in the antioxidant polyphenols lycopene, phytobene and phytofluene, has been shown to reduce blood pressure for treated but not completely controlled hypertensive individuals as well as never-treated men and women in the category of pre-hypertension. Two studies have been carried out at the University of the Negev, in Beer Sheva, Israel, by Dr Esther Paran and her colleagues.

Published in the *American Heart Journal*, the first study involved 31 men and women who had not taken anti-hypertensive drugs but had been diagnosed as having higher than normal blood pressure. This was a placebo-controlled study in which the patients were given a single daily dose of a commonly available tomato extract product, Lyc-O-Mato, containing 15mg of lycopene, 1mg of phytofluene, 1mg of phytotobene and the antioxidants beta-carotene and vitamin E. No other supplements were allowed.

Participants in the study included adults aged 30 to 70 years of age whose blood pressure was between 140–159 mmHG systolic and 90–99 mmHG diastolic. For the first four weeks, they took a placebo and their blood pressure was monitored and recorded. Then they took the Lyc-O-Mato tomato extract for eight weeks, after which they returned to another month of placebo capsules. During the treatment period, average systolic blood pressure readings fell from an average of 144 to 134 mmHG while average diastolic declines went from 87.4 to 83.4 mmHG. That drop of 10 systolic and 4 diastolic is about as much as single anti-hypertensive drugs can achieve. A significant improvement was noted after the first six weeks of taking the extract and continued through the entire eight-week test period. No improvements occurred during the placebo stages, with BP returning to pre-treatment levels when the placebo replaced the extract. There were no changes in weight or physical activity during the study. The only factor operating in the BP improvements was the tomato extract.

The aim of the second Israeli study with tomato extract was to evaluate the potential change in systolic and diastolic BP in treated but uncontrolled hypertensive patients after an eight-week treatment period. Dr Paran and her colleagues also studied changes in nitric oxide during treatment. This was the gold standard of medical research: a randomised, double-blind, cross-over, placebo-controlled study. 'Double-blind' means that neither doctor nor patient knew whether the pill contained the active agent or a placebo 'sugar pill'.

Fifty-four subjects were chosen whose blood pressures remained raised despite the use of anti-hypertensive drugs. Often two or three different drugs are required to completely control hypertension, but such combinations frequently lead to side effects that commonly limit compliance with doctors' prescriptions. Dr Paran hoped that the tomato extract would offer an alternative to adding another drug or two.

Patients were aged from 30 to 70 years of age and did not have other medical problems. After a routine baseline evaluation to determine weight, blood pressure and blood values, including cholesterol, study participants entered two double-blind, cross-over treatment periods of six weeks each, with either daily tomato extract (Lyc-O-Mato) or a placebo. Neither the doctors nor the patients knew who was taking which and, following the first phase, the groups were 'crossed over' so those previously on a placebo received the tomato extract and vice versa.

During the study, both blood pressure readings and levels of nitrate – the metabolite or breakdown product of nitric oxide – were measured and recorded. NO levels were significantly increased and blood pressure averages dropped by 8–11 mmHG systolic and 3–5 mmHG diastolic. That's about what doctors would hope for in adding a second anti-hypertensive prescription drug.

Previous research with the DASH study (Dietary Approaches to Stopping Hypertension) showed that increasing fruits and vegetables and wholegrains in the diet for eight weeks could lower blood pressure with average reductions of 2.8 mmHG systolic BP and 1.1 mmHG diastolic. Compare those numbers with the improvements with tomato extract! Could one simply choose to increase tomato consumption? Perhaps, but one Lyc-O-Mato capsule is the equivalent of eating *four* tomatoes daily, and those tomatoes would have to be cooked to release the lycopene for best bioavailability.

No doubt there will be more research data with lycopene and tomato extract in the future. It may be, for example, that there would be a dose-dependent effect. That is to say, increasing the dose may yield even better results. As one example of how, in this case, more may be better, research has shown that a dose of 60mg of lycopene daily reduced LDL cholesterol by 14 per cent. Dr Paran pointed out to me via e-mail that those with higher BP levels to begin with showed the most significant improvements. Could boosting the dose also help bring your BP down lower? Or might you be able to achieve a lower BP by combining lycopene tomato extract with one of the other 'Secret Weapons' mentioned in this chapter? As one anatomy professor once taught me, 'We're all as different on the inside as we are on the outside.' It certainly would be worth your while to experiment a bit. You have nothing to lose, since all these potent weapons have no potential for harm, and everything to gain.

Lyc-O-Mato is available throughout the UK. Check your local pharmacy or health food store. Or, for additional information, visit www.lycored.com.

Weapon number four – Pycnogenol

Pycnogenol has a wonderful tale of discovery all its own, going back literally centuries to the time of early exploration of North America. During his expeditions in Canada, searching for a north-west passage to China, Jacques Cartier found himself trapped in the frozen Hudson Bay in the winter of 1535. Having depleted supplies of fresh food, his men began to develop scurvy. Twenty-five had already died and 50 more were seriously ill when Cartier was offered help from Chief Domagaia, who prepared a 'tea' made from pine needles and bark that was drunk several times a day by the ailing men. Within one to two weeks, symptoms of scurvy subsided and the men recovered fully.

(As a side note, remember that the most frequently used drug, aspirin, was discovered by Native Americans who brewed the bark of the willow tree to treat aches and pains. Of course, they didn't realise that the brown tea they shared with early settlers contained what scientists came to identify as acetylsalicylic acid, more commonly known as aspirin. And it was only within recent decades that medical researchers have determined just how is that aspirin works its anti-inflammatory and painkilling wonders by altering hormone-like substances called prostaglandins.)

Going back to Pycnogenol, and how it helped Cartier's men fight scurvy, it took centuries to learn that the pine needles provided a small amount of vitamin C and the bark yielded vitamin C supercharging bioflavonoids, members of the polyphenol family of plant-derived substances. In fact, it was only in 1984 that scientists identified and quantified the 'ingredients' in Pycnogenol.

Today, Pycnogenol is obtained exclusively from a tree called the French maritime pine that grows in a 4,000-square-mile area of forest along the Bay of Biscay, bordered by the Atlantic Ocean, between the wine-producing district of Bordeaux to the north and the Pyrenees to the south. It is sold under a number of brand names throughout the world, and has earned a 'pedigree' of benefits that is truly remarkable, acting as an extremely potent antioxidant and stimulating the enzyme eNOS (endothelial nitric oxide synthase) to produce nitric oxide (NO) in the arterial linings from arginine. Ah, so now I'll bet you've already made the connection, and the reason why arginine and Pycnogenol are two of my 'Secret Weapons', working hand in hand with each other in the fight against high blood pressure!

Let's tie things together a little more tightly. Remember my explanation of how the ACE inhibitor drugs prescribed for hypertension work to reduce angiotensin-I converting enzyme? German and Hungarian researchers, working in collaboration in 1996, found that Pycnogenol has a dose-dependent ability to block ACE from raising blood pressure. Those with normal blood pressure wouldn't be affected at all. But those with raised BP owing to excessive levels of ACE will lower their BP. Anti-hypertensive drugs also increase levels of

NO in the endothelium, relaxing the arteries for better dilation and constriction, and thereby lowering blood pressure. Again, Pycnogenol provides that benefit. Between the two modes of action, Pycnogenol has been proven safe and effective in human clinical trials. Two of the Pycnogenol studies are particularly worth noting and demonstrate its value.

In 2001 investigators at the University of Arizona at Tucson did a 'gold standard' study of Pycnogenol and blood pressure. This was a randomised, double-blind, placebo-controlled, prospective, 16-week trial to see how well this potent antioxidant would work in modifying blood pressure in mildly hypertensive patients. Again, that's really important since so much emphasis today is being focused on numbers just higher than normal, recognising that those numbers are forecasts of future hypertension.

In this sort of 'gold standard' investigation, the patients were selected at random, hence 'randomised'. Again, it was 'double-blind', meaning neither doctor nor patient knew what was being given. 'Prospective' means that it took a look forward, rather than relying on reports of what had been done by the patients in the past. And it was long enough in duration to see real effects.

Eleven men and women received either 200mg per day of Pycnogenol or a placebo. Their blood pressures ranged from 140–159 mmHG systolic and 90–99 mmHG diastolic. After eight weeks, those getting the Pycnogenol were switched to the placebo and vice versa. The results were statistically significant. Average improvements lowered the systolic pressure to 133. The higher the BP to begin with, the greater the improvement.

A second investigation, published in 2004, looked into whether Pycnogenol could be used to reduce the dose of an anti-hypertensive drug. The 58 male and female patients in the study, averaging 57 years of age, had been put on a course of 20mg of nifedipine, a drug in the class of calcium antagonists. Over a period of 12 weeks, their blood pressure was monitored and recorded regularly, and subjects received either a placebo or 100mg per day of Pycnogenol. Depending on their BP readings, every two weeks nifedipine doses were adjusted to maintain lowered levels of pressure.

Most patients at the end of the 12-week study had normal blood pressure readings and were able to cut the doses of their drug literally in half, from 20mg per day to just 10mg per day by supplementing it with 100mg per day of Pycnogenol.

Now, here's the problem I have as a medical journalist who is also trained in medical physiology and research. I keep asking questions that have no answers because the particular study wasn't structured to resolve those questions. For example, what would have happened if the Pycnogenol dose was increased to 200mg per day, as was the case in the University of Arizona research? Would one see a dose-dependent response? Could those patients have been completely weaned off their prescription medications? Would the results have been even stronger if subjects had also been instructed to decrease alcohol consumption, to get more physical activity, to practise stress management, to lose weight, to incorporate other supplements such as arginine? Each of those, researchers quickly explain, introduces a variable. 'Teasing' out the effects of one thing from another becomes extremely time-consuming and expensive.

Pycnogenol is widely available worldwide. Shop for it at your local pharmacy or health food store. And you can find more information at www.Pycnogenol.com.

At this point let me reiterate: research with the polyphenols has only been going on since the mid-1990s. We're just at the frontiers of a 'brave new world' of alternative approaches to health maintenance in general and blood pressure control in particular. When I began to write and speak about oat bran and niacin back in the mid-1980s, we were in the same boat. Since that time, both of those approaches have been 'cast in bronze' as clinically proven ways to lower cholesterol. There's no doubt in my mind that over the coming years, the use of arginine and various polyphenolic agents, including grape seed extract, lycopene from tomato extract, and Pycnogenol will be mainstream.

Availability of all the 'Secret Weapons' will increase over time. While combination products may include one or other of these 'Secret Weapons', probably the best and most economical products will provide only one ingredient, such as Pycnogenol or MegaNatural BP grape seed extract. The best way to see where to find them is on one of the internet websites I've listed.

We're all different. We all respond differently to approaches and interventions. Just think about sodium. Some people are sensitive, some are super-sensitive and others are not sensitive at all. When it comes to getting blood pressure readings to optimal levels, one size does not fit all. This book provides a foundation programme that everyone should follow: get to optimal healthy weight, increase physical activity, definitely quit cigarettes, manage your stress as best you can, lower your blood sugar levels if you're diabetic or borderline, and improve your diet by eating far more fruits and vegetables and wholegrains while balancing your electrolytes in terms of less sodium and more calcium, magnesium and potassium. Even if you have perfect blood pressure, you and I and everyone else should follow that lifestyle to improve health in general.

Then do some personal experimentation. Start with arginine supplements, perhaps with one of the other 'Secret Weapons'. See how you do after a month or two. If you need a bit more 'horsepower', add another one of those agents. Or, if you're like me, and want the best of all worlds, you can do exactly the opposite by starting with *all* the 'Secret Weapons' along with the lifestyle modifications. Perhaps you'd prefer to combine two of the agents. Again, see how well you do.

Eventually, as you see what works best for you, you can add or subtract one or another agent. With one of those inexpensive home monitoring devices, it's really easy to test yourself without having to go to the GP's practice, as one would have to do when the goal is cholesterol control – there's no way you can test your cholesterol levels at home.

One thing is absolutely and positively true. If you follow the recommendations I've been detailing in this book, you're definitely going to feel better, sleep better, enjoy life more and see your blood pressure come down. That should bring a smile to your face! And with that happy thought, I'll end this chapter with a sweet – quite literally sweet – way to further improve your blood pressure.

Chocolate and cocoa and your heart

Yup, it's really good for you, your heart, and your blood pressure. Lurking in the dusty medical libraries are about 150 articles published between 1996 and 2005, all extolling the benefits of chocolate and cocoa. How sweet is that? One such study came from the University of L'Aquila, in Italy, where researchers have been busily looking into the cardiovascular benefits of the flavonols, a type of polyphenol, found in cocoa products. Dr Claudio Ferri and his colleagues, in collaboration with investigators at Tufts University, in Boston, learned that flavonol-rich dark chocolate reduces blood pressure both during the day and night in patients with hypertension.

Not surprisingly, much of the research on cocoa has been done in the Netherlands, a country famous for its hot cocoa. A study of elderly Dutch men indicates that eating or drinking cocoa is associated with lower blood pressure and reduced premature mortality. Interestingly, the reduction in death rate was *not* associated with lower blood pressure. The researchers speculate that cocoa's rich content of bioflavonoids, potent antioxidants, may be responsible for that very desirable benefit.

Similar flavonols abound in fruits, vegetables, red wine and green tea. But chocolate products have a higher total flavonol content on a weight for weight basis. Please pay close attention to that. It means that a 100g dark chocolate bar has more of those polyphenols than 100g of, say, a serving of fruit. Now, you're not going to substitute the recommended five or more servings of fruits and vegetables with five or more chocolate bars! But, as I'll show you, you can get all the goodness of chocolate and cocoa without the fat and calories.

Another nice thing about the flavonols in cocoa is that they're absorbed very rapidly into the bloodstream. That might well explain why sipping a nice warm cup of cocoa before bedtime can quickly relax you for a good night's sleep.

Dr Ferri's group has reported that dark chocolate, but not white chocolate, reduces blood pressure in the healthy subjects they worked with. Then the Willy Wonka doctors wondered whether dark chocolate could actually lower BP in those with hypertension. They recruited 20 patients who had never been treated for their raised BP, which was from 140–159 mmHG systolic and 90–99 mmHG diastolic, and 15 similar individuals who had normal blood pressure readings. All subjects avoided red wine and green tea during the study period.

All the participants received either 100g per day of dark chocolate, estimated to contain 88mg of flavonols or 90g of white chocolate, devoid of flavonols, daily for 15 days. Then the groups switched the type of chocolate they received. The results were, to say the least, impressive. Systolic BP fell by 11.9 mmHG and diastolic BP came down by 8.5 mmHG for those eating the dark chocolate, while those consuming white chocolate showed no difference. That's a *huge* improvement, comparable to what you might get from a prescription drug. The blood pressure reductions persisted throughout both day and night. And as a special bonus, LDL cholesterol counts tumbled down by 10 per cent.

The chocolate used in the study was not only the dark – or 'plain' – variety, neither white nor milk chocolate, it was specially prepared to contain a very high level of cocoa flavonols. White and milk chocolates have either little or none of the beneficial flavonols.

How does cocoa spin its magic spells on blood pressure? Once again, it comes down to improved levels of NO in the blood, relaxing the arteries and making them more compliant. In an editorial accompanying the article published in *Hypertension*, it was suggested that the mode of action might involve inhibition of ACE, once again like those anti-hypertensive ACE-inhibitor drugs. Let's see: would I rather enjoy some cocoa or take a prescription drug? Hmm... As I sit at my computer at this very moment, I'm sipping a morning cup of coffee heavily laced with ultra-rich cocoa. More about that a bit later but first let's review more of the research.

Though the Aztec Indians of Mexico and Central America 'invented' cocoa, which was reserved for royalty, when one thinks of cocoa, thoughts of Holland come to mind. That's where much of the world's finest cocoa comes from, and cafés and restaurants in the Netherlands offer hot cocoa as a matter of course. So it's fitting that a fascinating investigation carried out by the National Institute for Public Health and the Environment in that country followed 470 Dutch men over a 15-year period. The volunteers were aged between 65 and 84 and were medically examined and interviewed about their diets every five years.

Over the course of the study, 314 men died, with 152 of those deaths from cardiovascular disease. Scientists determined that those who had consumed on average 4g of cocoa per day, about what you'd get in a few squares of dark chocolate, had significantly lower blood pressure than those who did not. But here's the real winner: they were also half as likely as the others to die from cardiovascular disease. And those with a really high cocoa consumption were less likely to die of *any* cause. No wonder those Aztec chiefs kept it to themselves!

Now back to examining some of the delicious research findings. An international team of investigators from the US and Germany further determined that the particular flavonol in cocoa is called epicatechin, not that that titbit of information is of particular value other than to chemists reading this book. What *is* of value is their finding that a flavonol-rich cocoa drink increased vasodilation of arteries, increased NO production, and boosted microcirculation. All those things contribute to lowering blood pressure.

Although the Aztec Indians are long gone from Mexico and Central America, other indigenous peoples have perpetuated the delicious habit of drinking cocoa. In fact, many of the Kuna Indians on Panama's offshore islands routinely slurp three to four cups of cocoa daily. It's pretty important to note that their blood pressure barely rises as these people age and that cardiovascular disease in general is rare. Maybe it's a matter of fortuitous genetics? When the Kunas move to the mainland, they lose their cocoa-drinking habits and both blood pressure and incidence of heart disease increase. When scientists examined the island-dwelling Kunas and their mainland counterparts, they found that islanders have six times higher levels of that flavonol epicatechin and double the amount of NO in their blood. And cocoa powder and cocoa extracts have been shown to have higher antioxidant capacity than many other flavonol-rich foods, including both green and black tea, red wine, garlic, blueberries and strawberries, although we all should include plenty of those foods in our diets as well. Man cannot live by cocoa alone. But it's a pretty good start!

As a side note, I've advocated a lot of heart-healthy foods over the decades that I've been a heart-health warrior. But not everyone is as crazy about fish as I am. Many find oat bran pretty boring. And it takes a lot of persuasion to get folks to really boost their fruit and vegetable consumption. Then we come to cocoa.

Who doesn't like or even love chocolate and cocoa? The Aztecs were correct when they thought of cocoa as a gift of the gods. But they didn't munch on chocolate candy bars all day. They drank their cocoa, and that's what I'd like to suggest that you do as well.

Much of the research on chocolate and cocoa has been sponsored by the Mars company. They have two things in mind. First, they'd like to boost their sales across the board and have introduced specially formulated dark chocolate bars branded as CocoaVia. But please don't think of those confections as health food. To get a beneficial dose of flavonols, you'd need to munch two bars daily. That will add about 200 calories a day, which, if not offset by increased physical activity or decreased intake of other foods, would lead to a weight gain of 9kg in the first year! And those bars would provide 36 per cent of the maximum amount of saturated fat in a heart-healthy diet. Not a good idea. Read the ingredients list of confectionary bars like that and you'll see what I mean. And prepare for an onslaught of advertising and promotion for the dozens of 'healthy' chocolate bars launched worldwide since 2006. The other motivation for funding research by the Mars company is the desire to isolate and 'package' the active flavonols to be sold either as an over-the-counter supplement or a prescription anti-hypertensive drug. To think that you can get something that powerful and good for your heart, today, not some time in the distant future, in a chocolate bar or a cup of cocoa.

On the other hand, savouring a couple of squares of a dark, rich chocolate bar now and then wouldn't be too bad an idea. If nothing else, doing so might teach you how to take a tiny bite at a time and allow it to melt on your tongue, fully enjoying the indulgent moment. But doing so should be a treat, not a daily habit. As time goes on, I'm noticing an increase in chocolate confections that tout their concentrations of cocoa, and that's a good thing, indeed. You'll find that even one little square can be remarkably satisfying.

Conversely, there's no need to limit your potential enjoyment of cocoa in many ways.

I mentioned that, as I've been writing this section, I've been sipping a cup of coffee laced with dark, rich cocoa. Nothing could be simpler. Just put a heaped tablespoon (yielding about 5g or more of pure cocoa) into a cup or mug and pour in the hot coffee. Sweeten with sugar or an artificial sweetener to taste. Perhaps splash in a dollop of milk. Enjoy! If you find you like this a lot, as I do, you can even add the cocoa powder to the ground coffee beans as you make your pot in the morning or any time of the day.

At the end of a long, often stressful day of work, I love to prepare a steaming cup of hot cocoa to sip while reading a book or watching a little TV before bed. Just the process of preparation starts the relaxation process, I guess because I know what's in store for me. This doesn't take culinary genius. Get out one of your favourite mugs. Spoon in a heaped tablespoon of dark cocoa and some sweetener (you'll definitely need to sweeten it, since pure cocoa is actually quite bitter). While doing that, you'll have some skimmed or semi-skimmed milk warming on the stove or in the microwave. Pour the steaming milk over the cocoa and sweetener, stir, and bring the mug to your nose as you would a fine glass of wine. Sit, sip, relax and mellow out. You and I both deserve a nice reward at the end of a long day. And this treat will actually lower your blood pressure when enjoyed regularly.

And there are many other ways to enjoy cocoa as well. Here's a cooling suggestion for a hot summer's day. Put a dollop of cocoa powder, a fairly ripe banana, a tablespoon of honey and a large glass of milk in a blender and swirl it into a delicious treat that'll also provide you with the BP-fighting electrolyte minerals calcium and potassium. I also like to spoon a generous heap of cocoa powder into the breakfast smoothies I've become virtually addicted to. Take a look at my suggestions in the recipe section (see page 292).

Depending on the time you have available, your lifestyle and inclination, think about making some cocoa desserts. Imagine truly healthy, therapeutic taste treats. Who doesn't love brownies? Or biscuits? I've spelled out some recipes at the end of the book.

But when shopping for cocoa powder, be careful. Read those labels! You *don't* want ordinary cocoa mix, the kind that you simply mix with water. Those are loaded with sugar and some of the worst possible fats, the partially hydrogenated oils along with powdered milk. Instead, look for packets and tins of pure, unadulterated cocoa powder. There are dozens of brands through the world. One of the most famous and popular is made by Droste, in Holland. One tablespoon, containing 5g of cocoa and nothing but cocoa, has a mere 15 calories. Green & Black's Cocoa Powder is another delicious choice. Go on an exploratory cocoa shopping trip to a few markets and pick up a few different brands. You'll find subtle differences in taste and piquancy.

Special note to readers

As you've read, early research shows great promise for these 'Secret Weapons'. In the coming months and years we can expect additional investigations and knowledge will grow. I'd suggest that, from time to time, you visit my website, www.thehealthyheart.net, where I'll post the latest developments, new products and cutting-edge information.

Chapter 15

Prescription Drugs: the Last Resort to Lowering Blood Pressure

Hypertension affects about one billion people worldwide. The higher the blood pressure, the greater the risk of heart attack, heart failure, stroke and kidney disease. Hypertension remains one of the Western world's major killers. Those facts cannot be denied. It follows then that the more one can lower blood pressure, the greater the reduction in risk.

For many, if not most, men and women, following the programmes and suggestions in this book will very effectively lower BP. In fact, the BP-lowering effects can be similar to, if not even better than, those of potent prescription drugs, when followed faithfully.

So why would I even bother to include a chapter dealing exclusively with those prescription drugs? There are two reasons. First, there are individual cases of hypertension that are so severe and life-threatening that one must use every option available. The person with a blood pressure of

225/115 mmHG is in immediate danger and must be given urgent attention. In such instances, prescription drugs may be unavoidable and I would be wrong to argue against their use.

Second, not everyone is willing to make the lifestyle modifications I advocate and to take the non-drug supplements I personally take and recommend. It truly troubles me to think about and admit it, but many would rather 'take a pill' prescribed by the doctor rather than to take personal responsibility. To make a comparison, dramatic cholesterol reductions are possible without the use of prescription drugs, but the cholesterol-lowering statin drugs remain best-sellers, making fortunes for the pharmaceutical companies.

If I were diagnosed with hypertension, I would ask my doctor to allow me to have a trial period of lifestyle modification and supplements as detailed throughout this book. I know from the experience of my own fight against cholesterol that I would do my utmost to succeed in that trial. Unless my initial BP was so high that even with my best efforts it remained at a dangerous level, I'm confident that the trial would be successful. But if I was starting with a degree of hypertension that, though lowered through such efforts, still posed a threat to my health, I'd very definitely work with my doctor to find a drug or drugs that would lessen or eliminate the risk.

In the worst-case scenario, maximising those lifestyle modifications and adding the BP-lowering supplements would still have tremendous benefits, even if I had to take one of those drugs. Simply enough, I would be able to minimise the dose needed and thus limit the potential side effects and adverse reactions that universally plague anti-hypertensive drugs.

Never forget that you are in partnership with your doctor and that you have a say in the decision-making process and that ultimately you will play a major role in your own health destiny. It is ironic that people will be more selective in working with a garage mechanic than with a doctor! You owe it to yourself and to your loved ones to find a doctor with whom you can establish an excellent personal relationship. Does your doctor answer your questions fully, consider your special needs and problems, and leave you with a sense of confidence? If not, find another doctor! If you have hypertension, controlling that condition will be a lifelong endeavour. And if you require anti-hypertensive drugs, a great deal of effort will go into the search for just the right drug for you and the proper dose. You'll be spending quite a bit of time with your doctor, so you'd better have a very good relationship with him or her!

The best patient is a well-informed patient. You need to know as much about your disease and potential therapies as possible. The world of anti-hypertensive drugs can appear bewildering at first. Having some knowledge about those drugs, and that doesn't mean that you need to become a pharmacist, will help both you and your doctor successfully lower your blood pressure. So let's begin with a brief survey of the drug categories and how those medicines work.

Categories of anti-hypertensive drugs and their side effects

Diuretics

The diuretic drugs lower blood pressure by helping the body to eliminate excessive fluid and sodium through urination. These are among the oldest and best established of all anti-hypertensive drugs. They are particularly effective for those who are sodium sensitive, individuals with a culturally high salt intake, and Afro-Caribbean people. Diuretics are frequently prescribed as 'first line' drugs and may be combined with one or two other BP-lowering drugs. Certain diuretics, the thiazides, can act as vasodilators, opening blood vessels. Doctors may also suggest a high-potassium diet or prescribe potassium supplements, since diuretics may bring potassium levels too low.

Side effects include weakness, leg cramps, fatigue, (infrequently) gout, increased blood sugar especially for those with diabetes and reduced libido and/or impotence. Frequent need to urinate can be annoying. Within the group, there are three sub-categories:

Thiazide diuretics (trade/brand name)
Bendroflumethiazide (generic)
Cyclopenthiazide (Navidrex)
Chlorothiazide (Diuril)
Chlortalidone (Hygroton)
Indapamide (Natrilix)
Metolazone (Metenix 5) (Not typically used for blood pressure control but rather as a very powerful diuretic for patients with refractory heart failure.)
Xipamide (Direxan)

Loop diuretics (trade/brand name)
Bumetanide (Burinex)
Furosemide (Lasix)
Torasemide (Torem)

Potassium-sparing diuretics (trade/brand name)
(This category is not usually used for blood pressure control)
Amiloride hydrochloride (generic)
Triamterene (Dytac)

Beta-blockers
The beta-blocking drugs, fully termed beta-adrenoceptor blocking drugs, slow heart rate and the amount of blood pumped, thus lowering blood pressure. They are routinely prescribed to patients following a heart attack (myocardial infarction or MI), since research has shown that taking these

drugs for at least one year after an MI can help prevent a second event. Beta-blockers are also used to treat heartbeat disturbances called arrhythmias. They work by blocking the effects of heart-stimulating substances such as adrenaline, as well as by decreasing production of adrenaline in the brain. Therefore they have a 'central mediating' effect on blood pressure. These drugs are often used in combination with other anti-hypertensive agents.

Side effects include reduced exercise capacity, lethargy, fatigue and impotence. People with diabetes must have their insulin responses monitored regularly.

Beta-blockers (trade/brand name)
Acebutolol (Sectral)
Atenolol (Tenormin)
Bisoprolol fumarate (Cardicor, Monocor)
Metoprolol tartrate (Betaloc, Lopresor)
Nebivolol (Nebilet)
Nadolol (Corgard)
Propranolol hydrochloride (Inderal)
Sotalol hydrochloride (Beta-Cardone, Sotacore)
Timolol maleate (Betim, Moducren, Prestim)

Generic versions are available too.

ACE (angiotensin-converting enzyme) inhibitors
By blocking the action of the enzyme that 'activates' angiotensin, which is involved with blood pressure control within the arteries, the ACE inhibitors prevent constriction of those blood vessels, instead causing dilation of those vessels and thus decreasing resistance to the flow of blood, which, in turn, lowers blood pressure.

Side effects may cause a skin rash or other allergic reactions, loss of taste, a chronic dry cough and possibly kidney damage. That said, ACE inhibitors are generally well tolerated.

Ace inhibitors (trade/brand name)
Captopril (Capoten)
Enalapril maleate (Innovace)
Fosinopril (Staril)
Lisinopril (Carace, Zestril, Caralpha, Lisicostad, Zestoretic)
Moexipril hydrochloride (Perdix)
Perindopril erbumine (Coversyl)
Quinapril (Accupro)
Ramipril (Tritace)
Trandolapril (Goptin, Odric, Tarka)

Generic versions are available too.

Angiotensin-II receptor antagonists (blockers)
These rather new drugs, commonly referred to as ARBs, block the hormone responsible for constricting arteries and for making the kidneys retain more sodium and water. The action is similar to that of the ACE inhibitors, but instead of lowering levels of angiotensin-II by blocking the needed enzyme, the drugs keep the chemical from having negative effects on the heart and arteries. ARBs are frequently prescribed for patients who develop a cough from taking ACE inhibitors.

Side effects include headache, dizziness and fatigue.

Angiotensin-II receptor antagonists (trade/brand name)
Candesartan cilexetil (Amias)
Eprosartan (Teveten)
Irbesartan (Aprovel)
Losartan potassium (Cozaar)
Telmisartan (Micardis)
Valsartan (Diovan)

Generic versions are available too.

Renin inhibitors

Renin inhibitors are entirely new drugs that target the renin-angiotensin system at the first step of the metabolic process that affects blood pressure in the kidney. By limiting renin, less angiotensinogen and hence less angiotensin is produced and blood pressure is beneficially affected. Authorities believe that this drug can also help to protect the kidney itself. Doctors are pretty excited about this drug made by the Novartis pharmaceutical company under the trade name Rasilex (aliskiren). It is not currently available in the UK.

Rasilex is a very potent and effective anti-hypertensive drug, based on clinical trials that have been conducted in the US, the UK, and elsewhere. It can be used alone or in combination with other drugs or with the 'Secret Weapon' supplements, if additional blood pressure reduction is necessary or to reduce dose. Currently, Rasilex is the only drug in the renin inhibitor class; additional agents will probably not be available until approximately 2012.

I am particularly interested in Rasilex and am delighted to see its availability for men and women with very high blood pressure who may not respond adequately to the 'Secret Weapons' alone or even with other drugs. Rasilex does not affect physiological and biochemical responses that are responsible for the dry cough, oedema and fluid build-up often associated with ACE inhibitors.

Talk to your doctor about whether this new drug might be helpful in your particular case and how you might use it in conjunction with the programme of this book.

Calcium-channel blockers

This category of anti-hypertensive agents, also called calcium antagonists, interrupt the passage of calcium into heart and arterial muscle cells. This widens the arteries, improving blood flow, and thus lowering blood pressure. Doctors also prescribe calcium-channel blockers to treat heartbeat irregularities and the chest pain of angina.

Side effects include heart palpitations, swollen ankles, rash, constipation, headache and dizziness. Different drugs within the category may be more likely to cause a particular side effect than another. Ask your doctor about this if he or she prescribes one of the following drugs.

Calcium-channel blockers (trade/brand name)
Amlodipine (Istin)
Diltiazem hydrochloride (Tildiem, Adizem, Angitil, Calcicard, Dilcardia, Dilzem, Slozem, Viazem, Zemtard)
Felodipine (Plendil)
Isradipine (Prescal)
Lacidipine (Motens)
Lercanidipine hydrochloride (Zanidip)
Nicardipine hydrochloride (Cardene)
Nifedipine (Adalat, Adipine, Cardilate, Coracten, Fortipine, Hypolar Retard, Nifedipress, Nifopress Retard, Slofedipine, Tensipine)
Nimodipine (Nimotop)
Nisoldipine (Syscor)
Verapamil hydrochloride (Cordilox, Securon, Univer, Verapress, Vertab)

Generic versions are available too.

Alpha-adrenoceptor blocking drugs
This group of drugs, also known as alpha-blockers, selectively blocks particular blood chemicals that cause the arteries to constrict. Blocking them relaxes the arteries, allowing for improved blood flow and lowered blood pressure.

Side effects include lightheadedness or dizziness, sleepiness, increased heart rate or dizziness when standing up from a sitting or lying position, caused by a drop in blood pressure. This is termed postural (or orthostatic) hypotension.

Alpha blockers (trade/brand name)
Doxazosin (Cardura)
Indoramin (Baratol)
Prazosin (Hypovase)
Terazosin (Hytrin)

Generic versions are available too.

Combined alpha and beta-blockers (trade/brand name)
These drugs provide the benefits of both alpha and beta inhibition and are used for those who have suffered damage to the heart muscle from a heart attack.

The most common side effect is dizziness when standing up from a sitting or lying position, caused by a drop in blood pressure. This is termed postural (or orthostatic) hypotension. Adjusting the dose may help.

Carvedilol (Eucardic)
Labetalol hydrochloride (Trandate)

Generic versions are available too.

Central alpha-2 agonists
Also called centrally acting alpha agents, this category of drugs is very different from others in that they act in the brain where they switch off brain activity that causes the arteries to constrict.

Centrally acting alpha agents (trade/brand name)
Clonidine hydrochloride (Catapres, Dixarit)
Moxonidine (Physiotens)
Guanethidine monosulphate (Ismelin)

These drugs have the potential of causing severe mouth dry-ness, drowsiness or constipation. Most common side effects are sleepiness and sexual dysfunction. Side effects vary by drug within the category. But if you develop any of these side effects, don't stop taking the drug suddenly as your blood pressure could rapidly soar to dangerous levels. Speak to your doctor.

Methyldopa (Aldomet)

This drug may lower blood pressure so much that when you stand or walk you might feel weak or you may even faint. It can also cause sleepiness, sluggishness, dry mouth, fever, anaemia and impotence. Work with your doctor to adjust the dose and reduce those side effects as much as possible.

Generic versions are available too.

Arterial dilators (direct vasodilators)

As the name implies, these drugs open arteries by relaxing muscles in the wall of the vessels, allowing greater blood flow and reducing blood pressure.

Dilating drugs (Trade/brand name)

Hydralazine hydrochloride (Apresoline)

Side effects include headaches, swelling around the eyes, heart palpitations and joint pain or aches. These effects may lessen after taking the drug for a few weeks.

Minoxidil (Loniten)

Doctors typically reserve this potent drug for patients with extremely high blood pressure that has not responded to lesser therapies. It may cause water retention, leading to significant weight gain, and/or excessive hair growth. The company that developed the drug subsequently sold a greatly reduced dose as an over-the-counter treatment for male baldness.

Generic versions are available too.

Combination therapies

Most typically it will take two, three or even four different drugs, working in various ways as described above, to achieve adequate blood pressure control. Some drugs are available that combine two drug types, such as an ACE inhibitor and a thiazide diuretic, in one tablet or capsule. Some doctors like to offer their patients the convenience, while others prefer to customise the combination. The following are some of the combination drugs available.

Captopril and hydrochlorothiazide (Co-zidocapt, Capozide)
Enalapril maleate and hydrochlorothiazide (Innozide)
Irbesartan and hydrochlorothiazide (CoAprovel)
Lisinopril and hydrochlorothiazide (Carace Plus, Caralpha, Lisicostad, Zestoretic)
Losartan potassium and hydrochlorothiazide (Cozaar-Comp)
Quinapril and hydrochlorothiazide (Accuretic)
Telmisartan and hydrochlorothiazide (Micardis Plus)
Valsartan and hydrochlorothiazide (Co-Diovan)

British medical authorities got a lot of media attention when they proposed a 'polypill' that would combine a cholesterol-lowering drug and two blood pressure medications. Their rationale was that many patients have raised levels of both cholesterol and blood pressure, and so giving a single pill could potentially prevent many heart attacks, strokes and deaths. This particular combination isn't currently on the market.

In the US, one product combines atorvastatin for cholesterol lowering and amlodipine for blood pressure reduction. It is available in a wide variety of doses of both agents, allowing doctors to choose the one that would best suit a particular patient. That's much better than a fixed combination, since typically 'one size does *not* fit all'. It is not currently available in the UK.

So which drug is best?

That question might seem fairly straightforward, but it is highly controversial. In the UK, GPs no longer offer beta-blockers as a first treatment for hypertension. Black people suffering from high blood pressure and all those over 55 will receive either a calcium-channel blocker or a diuretic drug. Those under 55 will first be treated with ACE inhibitors. Some patients could get a combination of two or three different drugs, depending on the severity of their condition. These are the new guidelines issued by the National Institute for Health and Clinical Evidence (NICE) in conjunction with the British Hypertension Society in July of 2006 after reviewing available treatments.

According to Professor Bryan Williams, of University Hospitals NHS Trust, in Leicester, 'What we have found is that although beta-blockers remain effective at reducing stroke and heart disease, they are slightly less effective than alternative forms of treatment.'

Studies have been published and widely publicised with members of the medical community coming to very different conclusions. Some say always start with a diuretic and add other drugs as needed. Other doctors prefer to initiate therapy with an ACE inhibitor. Often cost is offered as a rationale. According to the Heart Foundation in Australia, 'Fewer than 50 per cent of patients treated for hypertension will achieve an optimal blood pressure response with a single agent (monotherapy). In the majority of cases a combination of anti-hypertensive drugs from two or more anti-hypertensive drug classes will therefore be required.'

One of the most cited studies, the Anti-hypertensive and Lipid-Lowering Treatment to Prevent Heart Attack Trial (ALLHAT), concluded that the thiazide-type diuretics are 'unsurpassed in lowering blood pressure, reducing clinical events, and tolerability, and less costly'. Results of that study, familiar to all doctors who treat hypertension, were published in 2002. The same conclusion was reached in 2006 by researchers at the University of Texas who noted the superiority of diuretics over calcium-channel blockers and ACE inhibitors in treating hypertension and preventing heart failure. It's worth noting that about two out of every three patients in ALLHAT needed two or more drugs to bring their BP down to below 140/90. Patients in that study were over 55 years of age and one-third were black. Both groups are most likely to respond to thiazide medications.

Literally dozens of studies have been published, often with varying conclusions. The Australian National Blood Pressure 2 study demonstrated the benefits of ACE inhibitors. That was also the case in the Heart Outcomes Prevention Evaluation (HOPE) study, which specifically worked with the ACE inhibitor ramipril.

Doctors look to the medical literature for guidance, but often find conflicting information and data. For example, a study funded by the US National Heart, Lung and Blood Institute found that diuretic drugs work as well or better than amlodipine in protecting against heart attack and stroke. The cost of a diuretic drug, widely available in generic forms, is a fraction of that of amlodipine.

Conversely, the much-touted ASCOT (Anglo-Scandinavian Cardiac Outcomes Trial) study found that treating with beta-blockers, diuretics or both increased the risk of developing diabetes by about 40 per cent and had some other side effects as well.

Certain population groups are also served better by

particular drugs. Those who are sodium sensitive and/or who are members of an ethnic group such as African-Americans/ Caribbeans whose diet is high in salt, will frequently do best with diuretics or calcium-channel blockers or both, studies have found and doctors have observed over the years.

The beta-blocker drug atenolol has long been viewed as sort of a 'gold standard' in anti-hypertensive agents and has been prescribed frequently by doctors as the one to start newly diagnosed hypertensive patients on. But studies of late have cast a shadow on atenolol, showing no particular benefit in terms of BP-lowering advantage and less-than-desired ability to prevent heart attack and stroke.

Patients most often have more than one medical problem at a time. For those suffering from heart (mitral) valve disease along with hypertension, ACE inhibitors seem to be a good choice. But not for those with valvular disease and normal blood pressure.

Diabetic individuals pose an entirely different challenge to doctors. They are at much higher risk of cardiovascular disease, and blood pressure targets for diabetics are significantly lower than for those without that disease.

Doctors also consider 'potentially unfavourable effects' of particular drugs on co-existing conditions:

Co-existing condition	Drug
Asthma	beta blockers
Low heart rate (bradycardia)	beta-blockers, calcium-channel blockers
Diabetes	beta-blockers, diuretics
Gout	thiazide diuretics
Heart failure	calcium-channel blockers, alpha-blockers
Kidney disease, pregnancy	ACE inhibitors, ARBs
Peripheral vascular disease	beta-blockers (atherosclerosis in leg arteries)

The United States and New Zealand are the only two countries that permit drug advertising by pharmaceutical companies. That's good for the UK and the rest of the world, but bad for those two countries. TV adverts provide often misleading information in the rosiest possible tones, promising great results without disclosing the full picture, and urge viewers to 'talk with your doctor' about this drug or that. Doctors often feel pressured by patients coming into the surgery with demands for that particular drug, putting the credibility of a 30-second TV spot or a magazine advert ahead of a doctor's medical training and years of clinical experience.

Ultimately the decision must be made by your own doctor, taking into consideration your unique medical history and patient profile. Assuming that you have confidence in your doctor – something I believe is essential – trust his or her judgement. But be sure to communicate effectively. Let your doctor know about any and all side effects that crop up. Remember always, however, that you must not abruptly stop taking any anti-hypertensive drug, since that could result in a severe change in blood pressure that could be very dangerous and possibly life threatening.

Conclusion

No single drug will completely cure hypertension. And no doctor will disagree with that. Proper treatment, if indeed drug therapy is needed, must also include aggressive lifestyle modification for best results. That includes weight control, moderation in alcohol consumption, cigarette cessation, increased physical activity and stress management. Without such efforts, the chances of attaining optimal blood pressure are greatly reduced. As my last thought in this paragraph, although prescription drugs for blood pressure control can have side effects, those are not experienced by all patients. Again, by working closely with your doctor you can have the best of both worlds: blood pressure control with the least possible adverse effects.

Chapter 16

The Blood Pressure Cure Express Programme

I've packed a lot of information about blood pressure and ways to control it into this book. But from time to time you may want to do a quick review or find the name and website of a particular supplement or some other detail. That's why I've put together this summary, a quick, express programme of the entire Blood Pressure Cure.

Blood pressure: definitions and testing

Blood pressure is a measure of the force of blood rushing through and pushing against arteries. Measured in millimetres of mercury (mmHG), systolic blood pressure, the top number in, say, 120/80, indicates arterial pressure as the heart beats while the diastolic, the lower number, is the pressure between beats, while the heart rests.

Raised blood pressure constitutes a major risk for cardiovascular disease, the number one killer of both men and women. As with high cholesterol levels, there are no symptoms of high blood pressure, or hypertension.

Ideally, blood pressure should be no more than 120/80 mmHG. When blood pressure increases to a range of 120–139/80–89, one is said to be in a state of pre-hypertension, a term originated in 2003. Men and women with pre-hypertension are at some increased risk of cardiovascular disease that could eventually lead to heart attack or stroke and are likely to see their blood pressure increase over the years unless they take steps to control it. A level of 140/90 mmHG or more is regarded as hypertension. The higher that blood pressure rises the greater the risk.

Blood pressure testing in a GP's surgery may be inaccurate owing to the anxiety of the patient or other factors. For a diagnosis of hypertension, doctors take measurements on three separate visits with patients seated with their feet on the floor, back supported in a chair and relaxed. Today's home blood pressure monitoring devices have been shown to be as accurate or more so than in a GP's surgery. A good brand to consider for your home is Omron; select one with a cuff that goes around the upper arm rather than the wrist for greatest accuracy. I believe that home monitors should be as common as bathroom scales.

Blood pressure and weight

Overweight and obesity predispose an individual to raised blood pressure. It is important to try one's very best to attain an ideal, healthy body weight. As a simple rule of thumb, men should have a waist circumference (WC), a belt size, no greater than 100cm (40in) and women no more than 80cm (32in).

Weight loss is not easy but it can be achieved. As a first step, keep a daily diary of everything you eat and drink for a week. Read your diary and determine what foods and beverages are contributing excess calories and where you can cut back. Consider what I call pre-emptive snacking. Enjoy small, healthy snacks throughout the day so you never get so hungry that you overeat. Before heading out to a restaurant or party, take the edge off your appetite so you'll eat smaller portions.

Blood pressure-friendly foods

Several studies have come to the same conclusion that those who eat the most fruits and vegetables, wholegrain bread and cereals, small amounts of lean meat, fish and poultry and fat-free or low-fat dairy foods are least likely to develop hypertension. And by adopting that eating pattern one can significantly lower blood pressure, by as much as one might expect from a prescription blood pressure drug. The most well known of those studies is termed DASH, for Dietary Approaches to Stop Hypertension.

Physical activity

The Greek physician Hippocrates said it hundreds of years ago, though in more elegant terms: move it or lose it! An essential part of a heart-healthy lifestyle involves physical activity. That doesn't necessarily mean going to the gym, jogging or other strenuous exercise you may not enjoy. The goal is a mere 30 minutes daily of simply moving around actively. That might mean taking a brisk walk, going dancing, gardening or any other activity. Another way to look at it would be to aim to walk 10,000 steps a day. You can do that with three ten-minute walks, taking the stairs rather than the lift or parking the car at the furthest end of the car park. Keep track of your daily steps with a good quality pedometer such as the Yamax Digiwalker (www.new-lifestyles.com).

Coping with stress

We all have some stress in our lives – in our work, in our personal lives and in ordinary, day-to-day activities such as driving in heavy traffic. All stress and anger raises the heart rate and blood pressure, and those rises can become permanent. We can't rid ourselves of all our stress, but we can learn to cope with it. One very efficient way is by increasing physical activity. Another is to take what I call mini-holidays. Take two minutes' break a few times a day, especially when stressed or angered, and simply close your eyes and concentrate on slow, rhythmic, deep breathing. Imagine your chest as a balloon you fill with air as fully as possible and then slowly deflate. RESPeRATE is a wonderful, clinically proven device to learn to control breathing, heart rate and blood pressure. Check it out at www.resperate.com.

Salt and sodium

We've heard a lot about how cutting back on salt and sodium is essential to blood pressure control. But take that advice with the proverbial pinch of salt! Yes, very high intake can raise blood pressure. And extreme restriction can lower it. But this approach isn't practical and many men and women are not sensitive to the effects of salt and sodium. By all means practise moderation. But most of the sodium in the modern diet comes not from the saltcellar or the salt on the rim of a margarita glass but, rather, from processed and tinned foods and from fast-food restaurants.

Along with moderation, we can counterbalance sodium by increasing our consumption of the other mineral electrolytes – calcium, magnesium and, especially, potassium. Aim for a daily intake of about 4,500mg of potassium by eating more fruits and vegetables and by adding a teaspoon or two of salt substitute consisting of potassium chloride when cooking. Enjoy fat-free and low-fat dairy products or consider a daily calcium and magnesium supplement. Mushrooms and shellfish offer a lot of magnesium. Or again, consider a supplement. Cal-Mag is a combination mineral supplement made by Endurance Products (www.endur.com).

Alcohol

Not long ago, doctors told patients who were battling with hypertension to avoid alcohol entirely. Today the word is 'moderation'. In fact, one to two drinks daily can actually improve blood pressure levels. One for women, two for men.

Don't forget cholesterol

Research shows us that as we reduce high cholesterol levels, blood pressure comes down as well. That's a nice bonus, fighting two risk factors at once. Limit saturated and trans fats in the diet. Eat a lot of fruits, vegetables and wholegrain bread and cereals. Enjoy plenty of the healthy fats, including olive and oils, nuts of all kinds, avocados and fish that provide heart-protecting omega-3 fatty acids. For those with a genetic predisposition to high cholesterol (80 per cent of all the cholesterol in the bloodstream is produced in the liver) a better alternative to statin drugs is larger-than-nutritional doses of the vitamin niacin that both lowers the bad LDL and raises the good HDL. Plant sterols called phytosterols are also proven to lower cholesterol; find them in supplements or in fortified foods (www.endur.com).

'Secret Weapons' against high blood pressure

Four supplements have been clinically proven to dramatically reduce blood pressure levels, producing results as good as would be expected from prescription anti-hypertensive drugs but without the side effects. Those four 'Secret Weapons' newly introduced to the market include:

- Sustained-release **Arginine**, an amino acid that helps the body produce a gas in the lining of the artery called nitric oxide (NO) that relaxes the artery, making it more elastic and flexible and thus allowing more efficient blood flow and resulting in lower blood pressure. Find **EP Sustained-Release L-Arginine** at www.endur.com for the best formulation at the most reasonable prices. Take three tablets in the morning and in the evening. Caution: ordinary arginine in health food stores won't produce the desired effects because it does not remain in the bloodstream.

- A specially formulated grape seed extract that concentrates the isolate clinically proven to bring blood pressure down is sold as **MegaNatural BP** by Polyphenolics. Take one capsule daily at any time. Find it at www.polyphenolics.com. Again, standard formulations of grape seed extract will not be expected to lower blood pressure.

- **Lyc-O-Mato** is a tomato extract that Israeli researchers found in two studies to lower blood pressure in patients who were currently taking anti-hypertensive drugs but were not at target levels and in patients who had never taken drugs for their raised blood pressure. The dose used in the studies was 15mg daily, either at once or in divided amounts. While it contains the powerful antioxidant lycopene, that substance alone does not lower blood pressure. Visit www.lycomato.com or www.lycored.com. You can also find it at www.vitaminshoppe.com, www.swansonvitamins.com, and www.healthyorigins.com.

- **Pycnogenol**, a particular formulation of French Maritime pine bark extract, has been proven also in human clinical studies to effectively lower blood pressure. Only that formulation has been tested, so other products containing pine bark extract may not necessarily work. The recommended dose is 200mg daily. To locate internet distributors of **Pycnogenol** go to www.Pycnogenol.com.

To start, I'd recommend taking the sustained-release arginine and one of the other 'Secret Agents'. Try them for six to eight weeks. If additional blood pressure reduction is needed, add one of the others. Or you could begin with all four and gradually cut back. Arginine in all cases should be the backbone of the effort, in concert with one or more of the others.

The fifth of my 'Secret Weapons' is a pure delight. Enjoy a relaxing mug of steaming, fragrant **cocoa** in the evening while winding down from the day, perhaps an hour or so before bedtime. Don't use the mixes that combine **cocoa** with sugar and various fats. Choose a brand of the darkest, richest **cocoa** you can find. The darker the **cocoa** the more polyphenols it contains, and it's the polyphenols that have been clinically documented to reduce blood pressure. Mix a heaped tablespoon of **cocoa** with 225ml skimmed milk and a sweetener of your choice, heat on the stove or in the microwave, and enjoy!

Best wishes for lower blood pressure and a healthy, happy heart!

Chapter 17

Delicious Recipes for Healthy Blood Pressure

I am not now, nor have I ever been, a member of the Food Police! Those are the health zealots whose food philosophy can be summarised simply as follows: if it tastes good, spit it out. I happen to love food. And I believe that truly delicious food can also be good for your health.

If you've travelled in Italy, Spain, the south of France, Greece or the Far East, you'll have enjoyed the wonderful native cuisines. Those foods happen to be some of the best in the world for heart health in general and for blood pressure control in particular. As an appetiser in Italy you might munch on bruschetta – crusty bread topped with olive oil, garlic, chopped tomatoes and basil. In Spain you might have a salad of roasted red peppers sprinkled with capers and a bit of crumbled cheese. How could you visit Marseilles in France without sitting down to a bowl of steaming bouillabaisse?

Then, if you're like most people, you'll have come home and returned to your old eating habits. Who'd think of making bruschetta? Or red pepper salad? Or bouillabaisse? Or any number of wonderful dishes that your heart would thank you for? Too much work, you might think. Not enough time to prepare. I hope to change your mind in this chapter, to share with you some of my favourite foods, and to show you how easy it is to enjoy a wide variety of heart-healthy foods on a regular basis.

Obviously, this is not a cookbook. I'd just like to give you some ideas that could perk up your taste buds while bringing down your blood pressure. And since the research data are so convincing that a diet rich in fruits and vegetables contributes to healthy blood pressure levels I'm going to stress those foods. I think you're going to surprise yourself by actually enjoying fruits and vegetables more than you thought possible. All I ask is that you give some of these ideas a chance.

I really believe that the reason both Americans and British people eat so little in the way of fruit and vegetables is because neither knows what to do with them beyond simply peeling a banana or boiling a bunch of carrots. Pretty boring for the most part. Sure, a nice ripe banana can be a quick, tasty snack. But very little effort converts that humble banana into a spectacular flaming dessert. And those carrots come alive with flavour after adding a touch of this and a sprig of that.

I also know that few of us have the time or inclination to follow complicated instructions in recipes. While I have an entire library of cookbooks, most of the time I cook without a recipe at all. I just throw a little of this and that together, spending as little time as possible. Sure, what I'm about to put into this book are 'recipes', but I'm hoping you'll use them as suggestions rather than following them to the letter.

Try to 'taste' the foods as you read about them. It's difficult to think about slicing into a juicy lemon without it making your mouth water. With a little practice you can accurately predict how a dish will taste when you prepare it. And if you see something in one of my suggestions that you dislike, simply avoid that ingredient. Conversely, if you see an ingredient you really like, you might want to double the amount I recommend. I do that most of the time when a recipe calls for garlic. No vampires in my house!

I'll start with a little story I like to tell about a cooking class my wife and I took at a French restaurant years ago when we lived in Chicago. The little bistro was owned and operated by a husband and wife, Renee and Josie, who both cooked and loved food. Josie stressed the notion of simply looking around at what you have in your kitchen and coming up with something delicious to eat.

As an example, one evening she took an orange and said it would be a good start for a dessert. She sliced off the rind, cut the orange into quarters, placed those slices on a plate, sprinkled them with a little brown sugar, and then drizzled some dark rum over the top to complete the delicious treat. Josie passed the plate around for us to taste, and the whole class loved it. There you have it: a recipe in just one sentence. You won't even have to pull this book out when you want to make this quick and easy dessert. You could even dress it up for company with a few sprigs of mint. Do you have young children in your family? Drizzle their orange with alcohol-free rum extract.

Some of the recipes in the coming pages will be just that simple, while others will have step-by-step instructions and lists of ingredients. But even those in that latter class will be so simple that after the first preparation you'll probably have memorised it so that you'll be able to throw it all together the next time.

I have not provided nutrition information for the recipes in this chapter. Why? None of the recipes contain the fats you should avoid. And all provide the nutrients essential for good heart health while being very low in calories. Don't worry about numbers. Just eat good foods.

Salads

Mediterranean/Greek Salad

With few variations, this is the staple salad whether you're in Greece or elsewhere in the Mediterranean. Start with a cucumber and a tomato, more than one each if preparing the salad for more than two or if you'd like leftovers. I prefer to peel the cucumber, though some folks don't. Or you could get fancy and run a fork's tines down the length to score the peel. One way or the other, slice the cucumber lengthways into quarters and then cut it into bite-size chunks. Do the same with the tomato. Mix with oil and vinegar or a bottled dressing of your choice. You can add a few sprigs of mint if you like – that's the way they do it in some countries. Chill in the refrigerator. Serve with crumbled low-fat feta cheese.

Tri-colour Roasted Pepper Salad

At first reading you might think this is complicated and difficult, but if you try it you'll not only love it but you'll also see how simple the salad is to prepare. Start with three peppers, red, yellow and orange. Cut off the tops, slice each in half, and remove the seeds and membranes inside. Flatten the pepper halves, arrange them on a grill pan, and place under the grill. Grill until the skins are completely blackened, remove, and place in a plastic bag for about an hour. By the time the roasted peppers are cool, you'll be able to remove the blackened skins easily. Rinse under running water.

Arrange pieces of the three peppers on salad greens on individual plates, drizzle some good olive oil over, scatter a few capers and a little crumbled feta or blue cheese over the top. Enjoy with a chunk of crusty bread. This is festive enough for company, a truly attractive dish, and something you can prepare an hour or so before your guests arrive.

Greens, Cheese and Peppered Honey Salad

The name says it all. To one side of each plate, pile some seasonal greens. On the other side of the plate, place a thin slice of cheese of your choice. It could be a low-fat mozzarella, feta or fontina. I use whatever happens to be in the refrigerator at the time. Dribble honey over both cheese and greens, and coarsely grind pepper over both. Or if someone in the family dislikes pepper, as my wife Dawn does, skip that for his or her plate, though I personally think the combined tastes of honey and pepper are a wonderful and delightful surprise. I enjoyed this salad first in a restaurant, where I paid $10 each, and thought, 'Hey, I can do this!'

Honeydew Melon and Avocado with Honey/Lime Dressing

To fully enjoy this salad, wait till honeydew melon is in season and most juicy, sweet and full of flavour. Arrange alternate slices of melon and avocado over a few leaves of romaine lettuce. Blend equal amounts of honey and lime juice (fresh juice tastes best, of course) in a measuring cup. The juice reduces the sweetness of the honey and makes a wonderful dressing for the salad. It's best if all the ingredients are chilled in advance.

Three-bean Salad

I think every family in America has a favourite recipe for this classic salad so frequently brought to summer picnics, but this is one I learned from a neighbour and I think it is the best. Draining and rinsing tinned beans greatly reduces the sodium content. Please get into that habit of this if you don't do so already.

65g granulated sugar
100ml rapeseed oil
175ml red wine vinegar
1 tsp salt
450g tin cut green beans, drained and rinsed

450g tin chickpeas, drained and rinsed
450g tin kidney beans, drained and rinsed
90g chopped red onions

Combine the sugar, oil, vinegar and salt in a large bowl. Add beans and onions and toss to coat thoroughly. Refrigerate in a large, covered container at least overnight. Stir once or twice, when you think of it, to develop the full flavour.

Red Potato Salad

Potatoes are great sources of potassium, and keeping the skins on preserves both fibre and nutrients in this recipe. Use whole eggs if you're taking phytosterols to block dietary cholesterol. Otherwise, you can use egg whites. I love this salad with hamburgers cooked on the barbecue during the summer.

2.2kg of red potatoes (pick the smallest ones)
2 medium green peppers (or one green and one red)
5 stalks of celery
12 large green olives with pimentos, sliced
12 hard-boiled egg whites or 6 whole eggs
Low-fat mayonnaise
Salt (optional)
Paprika

Boil the potatoes in (salted) water in their skins for about 15 minutes or till barely tender. While the potatoes cook, dice the peppers, celery and eggs. Allow the potatoes to cool, then cut into chunks. Mix all the ingredients with mayonnaise to taste. Sprinkle with paprika.

Sweet Potato Salad

Try this one for something different. It works really well with turkey roasted over the coals. Serve with cranberry sauce on the side. American Thanksgiving in the summer!

2 large sweet potatoes (yams)
100g diced celery (4 to 5 stalks)
100g diced apples
60g chopped walnuts
Low-fat mayonnaise
2 tbsp lemon juice
2 tbsp sugar
Salt (optional)

Cut the sweet potatoes into chunks with the skins left on to preserve the fibre and nutrients. Bring to the boil in (salted) water and cook until tender but not soft. While cooking the potatoes, prepare the other ingredients. When the potatoes are cool, mix all the ingredients with mayonnaise to taste.

Carrot Salad

0.5kg carrots, grated
90g sultanas
50g diced celery
1 tsp lemon juice
1 tsp granulated sugar
Low-fat mayonnaise

Nothing difficult about this one. Simply mix all the ingredients together with mayonnaise to taste. Grate the carrots by hand or with a food processor; or make it easy on yourself and buy grated carrots at the supermarket.

Colonel Kowalski's Coleslaw

This is my version of KFC's coleslaw. The trick is to chop the cabbage and carrots into tiny bits. I like the clean, crisp taste. It goes well with sandwiches of all sorts, adding the veggies we don't normally get at lunch. Chop, mix, chill and serve.

> 1kg chopped cabbage (use standard green cabbage or
>   half green and half red)
> 100g chopped carrots
> 100g granulated sugar
> Salt (optional)
> ¼ tsp ground white pepper
> 100g low-fat mayonnaise
> 100ml low-fat buttermilk
> 1½ tbsp white vinegar
> 2½ tbsp lemon juice

Hollywood Cobb Salad

I was lucky enough to move to Los Angeles just before the famous Brown Derby restaurant closed. The cobb salad invented there has been popular for decades because it's so delicious. I like it because it's one of the easiest ways to get plenty of veggies of all sorts. Make a big bag full and keep in the refrigerator.

> 200g chopped mixed greens
> 50g each: chopped mushrooms, broccoli, carrots
> 50g each: chopped sweet onions, beetroot, peppers

Combine all the ingredients and mix well in a large plastic bag. Keep chilled until ready to serve with the dressing of your choice. This recipe is enough for two people. Multiply the ingredients for larger groups or to keep on hand. Top the salad off with sliced grilled chicken or salmon and you have a complete, wonderful meal. Or put the chopped veggies in a sliced roll for a salad sandwich.

Soups to warm your soul and nourish your heart

Minestrone Soup

There are as many recipes for minestrone soup as there are Italian restaurants. Everyone has a favourite, and this is one of mine. Eat it in place of a salad at the start of a meal or have a large bowl for a satisfying meal with a chunk of crusty Italian bread and a glass of red wine. Please don't let the long list of ingredients put you off. You can't fail.

2 tsp olive oil
1 medium onion, chopped finely
1 spring onion, chopped finely
2 medium carrots, peeled and diced
2.25 litres low-sodium chicken stock
2 red potatoes with skins left on, diced
1 tin cannelloni or kidney beans, drained and rinsed
2 small courgettes, diced
2 celery stalks, diced
1 tin low-sodium whole Italian plum tomatoes,
   cut into chunks
1 tbsp tomato paste
½ small head of cabbage, chopped finely
½ tsp Italian seasoning
2 bay leaves
1 packet frozen spinach
Salt (optional)
½ tsp freshly ground black pepper
100g macaroni
75g frozen peas
3 tbsp chopped parsley (Italian broad leaf if available)

Place the onion, spring onion and olive oil in a large saucepan and sauté for about 3 minutes. Add the carrots and sauté for another 3 minutes. Add the stock and all the ingredients except the peas, parsley, tomatoes, spinach and macaroni. Bring to the boil, reduce the heat and simmer for one hour. Add the macaroni, tomatoes, spinach, peas and parsley and simmer for 10 more minutes. You'll find this is even more delicious the next day after all the flavours merge.

Jenny's Butternut Squash Soup

My daughter Jenny makes, I think, the best butternut squash soup you'll ever eat. This is definitely worth your while to prepare. Make enough for leftovers. Or make a double batch and freeze half for another time.

4.5kg butternut squash
350g chopped onion
2 tbsp olive oil
900ml low-sodium chicken stock
Salt (optional)
¾ tsp curry powder
¼ tsp each of ground nutmeg, white pepper, ground ginger
2 bay leaves
100ml low-fat sour cream

Preheat the oven to 180°C/350°F/Gas 4. Cut the squash in half and scoop out the seeds. Place the squash in a casserole dish, cut side down, in about 3cm (1in) water. Bake for 40 to 45 minutes. Allow to cool, then remove skin and cut into chunks. Meanwhile, place the onion in a medium-size saucepan, add the olive oil and sauté for about 3 to 4 minutes or until translucent. Stir in the chunks of squash, chicken stock and seasonings. Bring to the boil, then reduce the heat and simmer for 15 minutes. Remove the bay leaves and blend the soup in a food processor or blender in batches. Return to the saucepan, heat through and add the sour cream.

Cream of Vegetable Soup

This is a basic recipe for making any kind of cream of vegetable soup, simply choosing whichever vegetable(s) are in season or you'd like to use. This is a good example of how once you make it you'll never have to look at the recipe again. You'll just throw the ingredients together and it'll be done. Nothing to it at all.

        400g cauliflower/broccoli florets, asparagus, carrots or a
            blend of root vegetables
        900ml low-sodium chicken, vegetable or beef stock (try
            them all for variety)
        2 bay leaves
        ½ tsp ground white pepper
        ½ tsp tarragon
        ½ tsp thyme
        225ml low-fat sour cream

This is the essence of simplicity. Just put all ingredients in a large saucepan, bring to the boil, reduce the heat and simmer until the vegetables are very tender, almost mushy. Remove bay leaves. Allow to cool for easier handling. Blend in a food processor or blender in batches. Return to the saucepan and heat through. Blend in sour cream.

Greens and Stock

Every nutritionist says we should eat more leafy green vegetables such as endives, spinach and the like. But many people don't actually like greens very much. Instead of serving greens on the plate as vegetables, I like to make them into a simple soup. This isn't my invention, it's the way Italians have been cooking for decades.

Buy a bunch of greens at the supermarket and clean them under running water to get rid of any dirt and grit. Put them into a saucepan and pour in enough low-sodium stock (vegetable or chicken) to barely cover the greens. Flavour with some Italian seasoning and freshly ground pepper. Experiment with other herbs. Cook until greens are tender – that doesn't take too long, so don't go and read a book! Serve the greens in bowls as a side dish for the meal.

If you have a little more time and want to get fancy, start by sautéing two or three peeled garlic cloves in a tablespoon of olive oil until tender and translucent (never brown, since over-fried garlic turns bitter). Then add the greens and stock. When the stock comes to the boil, add half a tin of drained and rinsed cannelloni beans, heat through and serve. As the Italians say, 'Manje!'

Vegetable side dishes

Bruschetta

What we have here is a combination of bread and veggies. You can enjoy this as a starter before the meal or along with it. Make it once and it'll be as much a part of your cuisine as it is in Italy. And you'll laugh when you see it outrageously priced in restaurants.

Start with four large slices of good bread and toast them either in a toaster or under the grill. While they're toasting, peel four garlic cloves. Then run the cloves over the toasted bread. The bread will grate the garlic like sandpaper. Drizzle your best extra-virgin olive oil over the bread. Then top with chopped, seeded Italian plum tomatoes and finely chopped fresh basil leaves. That's it. Enjoy!

Acorn Squash

1 medium to large acorn squash for two persons
2 tbsp brown sugar
1 tbsp soft margarine

Cut the squash lengthways and remove the seeds and membranes. Pierce the flesh of the squash repeatedly with a fork, taking care not to cut through the skin. Use your fingers to smear the inside of the squash halves with margarine, then sprinkle on the brown sugar. Microwave for 12 to 15 minutes. Allow to cool for ease of handling, then use a tablespoon to remove the squash flesh from the skin and mix it with the margarine and sugar. Return the mixture to the skins and reheat in the microwave when ready to serve.

Roasted Root (and other) Vegetables

Don't you get sick and tired of just steaming or boiling vegetables? Of course you do. That's one of the major reasons why we don't eat enough vegetables. Here's an easy-to-do change of pace that you and your family will love. And so will your heart.

Let's start with the root vegetables that fill supermarkets in the autumn and winter. Peel four medium carrots, one parsnip, one turnip and one swede and cut into medium-size pieces. Place them all in a plastic bag, pour in 2 tablespoons of olive oil and sprinkle in a pinch of salt, some freshly ground pepper, and ½ tablespoon of tarragon. Mix well so the veggies are coated with the oil and seasonings. Arrange them in a single layer in an ovenproof casserole dish. Roast at 180°C/350°F/Gas 4 for about 15 minutes or until tender. (My wife likes her vegetables crunchier and I prefer mine cooked right through.)

You can use essentially the same technique for other vegetables as well. Asparagus is particularly delicious roasted in this fashion, as is broccoli. You can add some crushed garlic cloves to the asparagus. Also try beetroot. To roast potatoes, cut them into chunks with the skins still on and boil for a few minutes to soften them a bit before putting them in the oven.

Carrots and Dill or Parsley

Instead of buying beta-carotene supplements, eat more carrots and other yellow and orange vegetables such as squash. I'll bet you didn't know that beta-carotene is only one of more than 500 carotenoids found in carrots. Why settle for just one?

Start with a bunch of carrots. I like best the ones with the greens still attached. Don't worry about quantity, since leftovers are never a problem. Make plenty. Just peel the carrots (or simply scrub them with a clean brush under running water) and slice. Place the sliced carrots in a small saucepan and add just enough water to cover. Instead of adding salt to the water, add a heaped tablespoon of granulated or brown sugar. They taste so much better that way, and you get rid of some sodium in your diet. I also like to add ½ teaspoon of salt substitute to boost my potassium intake. Bring to the boil, and simmer until they're as tender as you like.

While the carrots are cooking, chop up 10g of fresh dill or parsley. Once the carrots are tender, drain the water, put in a tablespoon of margarine and the chopped herbs. You'll fall in love with carrots again.

(As a side note, I love the quote from famed chef and cookbook author Julia Child who said, 'If you don't want to cook vegetables till they're tender, eat crudités!' Crudités, of course, are raw pieces of veggies usually served with a dip as a snack or a starter.)

Roasted Tomatoes

This meal is rich in nutrients, simple to prepare, and absolutely delicious as a side dish with almost any meal. Simply slice a tomato or two in half, scatter a few shreds of fresh basil on each, and top with some parmesan cheese. Put the tomato in the oven for about 15 minutes or until the cheese is melted and the tomato is cooked through.

Lemon Broccoli

For this you will need about a half a kilo of broccoli florets for four persons. Place them in a shallow saucepan of water, bring to the boil, reduce the heat, cover and simmer until bright green and done to your desired tenderness. While the broccoli is cooking, mix the juice of ½ lemon (a little over 1 tablespoon), 1 tablespoon of olive oil, and a ¼ teaspoon of ground white pepper in a little dish. Drain the broccoli and drizzle over the lemon/oil mixture.

Sautéed Garlic Spinach

Here's a delicious way to get more of those leafy greens into the diet. You will need one bunch of spinach for a true-spinach lover who's really hungry or for two more typical persons. The most difficult part of spinach preparation is cleaning the leaves. I first rinse the bunch under running water to get rid of the dirt and grit, then put the leaves in a sink filled with cool water and swirl them around. Because I'm a fussy eater, I take the time to pinch off the stems so I get only the tender leaves. You could take the easy way out and simply buy a bag of pre-washed, pre-picked spinach – though I'd still recommend that you give it a quick rinse. Use a salad spinner or kitchen towels to dry the leaves. (They don't have to be bone dry.)

Peel and finely chop the garlic cloves. My wife and I love garlic, so I use 4 cloves per bunch. Put the chopped garlic in a fairly large saucepan with a lid and very gently sauté in 2 tablespoons of good olive oil, until the garlic is translucent. Don't let it brown, since that makes garlic bitter. Next, dump the spinach in the pan and cover. Put the pan on a very low heat for just a few minutes, tossing the pan now and then to make sure the spinach gets nicely coated with the garlicky olive oil. Serve and enjoy.

Simple Spinach

People often dislike spinach because it tastes bland. There's no reason for that.

Prepare the garlic and spinach as in the previous recipe. But don't bother to dry the leaves. Just dump the spinach in a large covered pot and cook over a low heat. The moisture on the washed leaves will be enough to steam the spinach.

Serve with a splash of balsamic or rice vinegar for a flavoursome treat. Or try something that my dad introduced me to: sprinkle the spinach with a little sugar. Sounds weird, but it's really good.

Green Beans with Tomato Sauce

This recipe is so good that my mouth is actually watering as I write it down even though I just finished breakfast. It's full of flavour yet simple to prepare.

> 0.5kg fresh green beans, cut into 5cm lengths
> 225ml low-sodium tomato sauce
> 1 tbsp olive oil
> 3 garlic cloves
> 1 tbsp parmesan cheese

Gently boil the green beans in a saucepan of water for about 8 minutes or until tender. (This would be another good time to add a ¼ teaspoon of salt substitute to get more potassium.) While the beans are cooking, peel and finely chop the garlic cloves, and sauté them in a pan with the olive oil. As soon as the garlic is translucent (but not browned) add the tomato sauce and heat through. Drain the beans, add the garlic tomato sauce, put on a serving dish, and sprinkle the parmesan cheese over the top.

Peppers and Sautéed Onions

Did you know that peppers, especially the yellow and red ones, have two to three times as much vitamin C as oranges do? They're also a pretty good source of potassium.

- 1 green and 1 yellow orange or red pepper, sliced into strips
- 1 medium sweet onion sliced
- 2 cloves of garlic
- 2 tbsp olive oil
- 1 tsp Italian seasoning
- ¼ tsp red cayenne pepper (optional if you don't like the 'bite' of pepper)

Sauté the garlic in olive oil in a frying pan until just translucent. Scoop out the garlic and reserve. Sauté the peppers and onions until tender. Add the reserved garlic, Italian seasoning and pepper and heat through. Colourful and delicious!

Grilled Aubergine

Ordinarily, I don't like aubergine very much. But I cooked this for Dawn because she loves the stuff. It was really good. Try this as an accompaniment to another grilled food, especially fish. That way you can prepare both at the same time.

Start with a large, firm aubergine – enough to serve four. Slice it lengthways and spread the following mixture on both sides of each slice with a brush:

- 2 tbsp olive oil
- 1 pinch each of salt and pepper
- ½ tsp Italian seasoning
- 1 clove of garlic, crushed
- 3 tbsp low-fat Italian dressing

If you want to take a short-cut, simply use regular Italian dressing that has olive oil as an ingredient. It won't be quite as good, but a bit easier. Now grill the aubergine slices for about 5 minutes on each side under a medium grill – just about the same amount of time you'd cook a piece of fish.

Cauliflower and Sultanas

Once again, cauliflower isn't one of my favourite vegetables. But that's when it's served raw as a crudité or simply boiled – boring and tasteless (in my humble opinion). This recipe bursts with flavour, and I prefer highly flavoured foods.

> 1 head cauliflower, cut into florets, leaves removed
> 175g sultanas
> 50ml gin (or rum or brandy or other spirits)
> 2 cloves garlic, peeled and minced
> 2 tbsp olive oil
> 1 tbsp balsamic vinegar
> 50g cup sugared walnuts or pecans

Start by soaking the sultanas in the gin or other spirits, making sure they're all covered. The longer they soak, the better. Prepare the cauliflower florets. Mix the oil, vinegar and garlic. Place the cauliflower in a shallow saucepan and just cover with water. (Here's another opportunity to add ½ teaspoon of salt substitute to the water to add potassium.) Cover and cook for about 3 or 4 minutes after the water comes to the boil or until barely tender to the fork. Drain off the water, remove the cauliflower and set it aside. Now add the oil, vinegar and garlic to the pan and heat it through before adding the cauliflower. Sauté just long enough for the garlic to become translucent. Mix in the nuts and serve.

Broccoli and Cheese Sauce

Here's another way to add wonderful flavour to a vegetable that's a fabulous source of potassium.

2 large heads of broccoli, cut into florets
100g grated low-fat cheddar cheese
100ml low-fat sour cream
25g each of finely chopped celery and onion
1 tbsp rapeseed oil
Pinch each of salt and pepper

Place the broccoli florets in a shallow saucepan and just cover with water. Bring to the boil, cover, reduce the heat to a low simmer and cook until bright green and tender without being mushy. Meanwhile, sauté the celery and onion in the oil until the onion is translucent. Mix the cheese and sour cream. Blend into the sautéed celery and onion and add the seasoning. Gently warm the mixture until the cheese melts. Drain the broccoli and place on a serving platter. Pour the sauce over. Get ready for compliments to the chef.

Simple Sweet Potato

A medium-size sweet potato with skin provides about 400mg of potassium. Why not include this tasty vegetable in your diet regularly? One way would be to make mashed sweet potatoes in the same way you would white potatoes. Even simpler, just poke a few holes in the sweet potato, pop it into the microwave for about ten minutes, and serve with a dab of margarine and another of low-fat sour cream.

Seafood

Fish in Foil

I especially love two things about this recipe. First, you can prepare it ahead of time so it's great for entertaining. Second, there are no pots or pans to clean up. It's also easy and fool-proof.

> 4 whole trout or baby salmon or other small fish (one
>   per person), gutted
> 1 onion sliced into thin rings
> 1 tomato cut into eighths and deseeded
> 2 celery stalks, chopped
> ¼ cup finely chopped parsley
> ⅛ tsp celery salt
> ⅛ tsp paprika
> 1 lemon
> Salt and pepper

Rinse the fish under cold water and pat dry. Place on a 30cm sheet of aluminium foil. Divide all the ingredients, except the lemon, and place inside the fish. Put aside any extra onion rings to place on the outside of the fish. Cut the lemon in half and squeeze the juice into the cavities of the four fish. Wrap and seal the fish in the foil. Indoors, bake for 15 minutes in a preheated oven at 190°C/375°F/Gas 5. On a barbecue, place the fish parcels in the middle of the grill and roast for 15 minutes.

Skewered Prawns and Scallops

Enjoy this recipe indoors in the oven or, as Aussies say, outdoors on the 'barby'. You can substitute chunks of fish for the scallops.

Marinade

  50ml chicken stock
  50ml rapeseed oil
  1 tbsp each: lime juice, lemon juice, orange juice and
    cider vinegar
  3 tbsp finely chopped parsley
  3 garlic cloves, peeled and chopped
  Pinch each of salt and pepper

Main ingredients

  200g of prawns
  200g of scallops or fish chunks
  2 peppers, one green and one yellow or orange
  1 medium onion cut into chunks
  4 small tomatoes, halved

Mix the marinade and pour into a plastic bag. Add the main ingredients and shake well to ensure they are covered with the marinade. Seal the bag and refrigerate for 2–3 hours. Skewer seafood and veggies alternately. Grill until prawns and scallops lose their translucency. Do not overcook these delicate foods.

Bouillabaisse

I got this recipe from a chef friend of mine who comes from the south of France but I have simplified it to save time. Yes, it still takes a bit of time and effort, but it's a great treat for a special occasion. You don't get much more festive than this. Serve with some crusty French bread and a chilled white wine.

> 500ml vegetable stock (or fish stock if available)
> 100ml fish stock
> 100ml white wine
> 2 bay leaves
> 2 celery stalks, chopped
> 1 fennel root, chopped (or ½ tsp each of fennel and anise seed)
> 1 large onion, chopped
> 3 medium carrots, peeled and chopped
> 4 garlic cloves, peeled and finely chopped
> ¼ tsp each rosemary and thyme
> ½ tsp orange zest (shavings of orange peel without the pulp)
> 6 whole black peppercorns
> 1 tsp salt (optional)
> 1 tsp salt substitute (for extra potassium)
> Around 0.5 kg assorted seafood of your choice, such as chunks of fish, prawns, clams or mussels, and perhaps crab or crayfish

There's quite a bit of controversy as to whether true bouillabaisse includes crustaceans but that's entirely up to you.

Place all the ingredients except the seafood in a large saucepan. Bring to the boil, and then reduce the heat and simmer for 30 minutes. Add the seafood and simmer for another 15 minutes.

Blackened Cajun Salmon

From France we go to French Louisiana, where Chef Paul Prudhomme created a dish that became a national favourite throughout the US. His original dish called for redfish, found in the Gulf of Mexico. But you can use salmon or other fish of your choice. This dish is spectacular for outdoors cooking as your guests watch the smoke billowing up from the barbecue. (Not a good idea to do this indoors unless you have a very efficient oven hood.)

Blackening seasoning
- 1 tbsp paprika
- 1 tsp garlic powder
- 1 tsp cayenne pepper
- 1 tsp onion powder
- 2 tsp salt (or one tsp salt mixed with one tsp salt substitute)
- ¼ tsp ground black pepper
- ½ tsp ground thyme
- ½ tsp oregano
- ½ tsp dried basil

250g salmon fillet (or other fish of choice) per person

Mix the seasoning ingredients together and set aside. This can be done any time in advance. (I make a large amount that I can use for several meals.) Now you'll need a cast-iron frying pan, large enough to accommodate all the fish, or you can do it in two or more batches. Place the frying pan directly on the barbecue coals or on top of a gas-powered grill and heat until literally white hot.

Meanwhile, rinse the fish fillets under running water and pat dry. Cover the fish fillets in the seasoning. Place a teaspoon or so of margarine on each fillet. Then carefully drop the fillets into the heated pan. Expect that billowing smoke! The fish will cook quickly owing to the high heat. After about 3 minutes, place another dab of margarine on the top of each fillet and flip with a spatula to cook the other side for about 2 minutes.

This is a spicy dish. (Many would say that's an understatement!) Serve with cold beer to soothe your tongue!

Smoothies – meals in a jug

I started drinking smoothies as a convenient way to have breakfast on my way to the golf course at weekends. Then I began to throw one together when I was in a hurry to get to a meeting in the morning. Now I keep a few jugs in my refrigerator and enjoy them throughout the week. The flavour combinations are virtually limitless, and so I never tire of them – and neither will you. This is an incredibly healthy habit to get into, since each smoothie contains three or four servings of fruit, many of which are excellent sources of magnesium and potassium, and skimmed milk provides both calcium and potassium. It's one of the best ways to balance your electrolytes, negating the effects of sodium in your diet.

One medium banana, a staple ingredient in all my smoothie recipes, has 470mg of potassium, cantaloupe provides 550mg per cup, a medium mango gives you 320mg, a medium pear has 200mg, 240ml of orange juice (or frozen concentrate to reconstitute to that amount) has around 440 mg and 240ml of grape juice offers 330mg. A 240ml serving of skimmed milk has 410mg of potassium along with 300mg of calcium. A smoothie made from milk, orange juice, a banana, a mango, and a pear would add up to a whopping 1,630mg of potassium! By the way, if you're looking for the potassium champion of the fruit world, that would be the durian (tastes like heaven, stinks like hell, they say) at 1,000mg per cup! That's not counting all the fibre and other nutrients. A smoothie of that size, typical of what I bring to the golf course, will satisfy you for most of the day until an afternoon snack or an early dinner.

I've included quite a few of my favourite recipes, frequently spiked with cocoa powder or grape juice concentrate to provide lots of flavour as well as a load of BP-healthy polyphenols. Add some berries to give you even more polyphenols. But there's no limit to the combinations of ingredients you can try.

On a happy, economical note, you'll never waste fruit when it gets a bit overripe! When certain fruits are in season, such as mangos and peaches, I buy them at their best taste and lowest price, let them get nice and ripe, and store in bags in the freezer. You can store bags of frozen fruits and berries, too. I also keep frozen orange and red grape juice handy. Egg substitute is an excellent protein source to balance the meal's nutritional profile. If your smoothie comes out thicker than you'd like, just add more milk or water or juice to thin it to your preference.

Preparation is simply a matter of putting all the ingredients into a blender and whizzing to a delicious mixture. I make two to three smoothies at a time for convenience and keep them in jugs in the refrigerator for when I need a quick meal on the go.

Basic Smoothie Recipe

240ml water (or orange juice if you have it)
240ml skimmed milk (80 calories)
60ml frozen orange juice concentrate (130 calories)
120ml egg substitute (60 calories) (never consume raw
  eggs owing to salmonella risk)
150g frozen mixed berries (70 calories)
1 medium banana (100 calories)
1 medium pear (100 calories)

Total calories: 530 (That's a very reasonable number of calories for breakfast or lunch.)

Creamsicle Smoothie

I've named this after a frozen confection of vanilla ice cream and orange sherbet on a stick that was very popular when I was a child and is still sold today – delicious and refreshing.

240ml water
240ml skimmed milk
60ml frozen orange juice concentrate
120ml egg substitute
1 medium banana
1 medium orange, peeled and seeded
1 tbsp honey
½ tsp vanilla extract

Fudgsicle Smoothie

Yup, named after another frozen confection on a stick. This one takes advantage of the high polyphenol content of plain cocoa powder (not hot cocoa mix).

240ml water
240ml skimmed milk
120ml egg substitute
1 medium banana
1 medium mango (replace with raspberries for variety and a special taste treat)
1 tbsp honey (more if you prefer it sweeter; you can also use artificial sweetener)
2 tbsp cocoa powder

Strawberry Screamer

I live in a part of California famous for strawberries. In fact, there's a strawberry festival every spring. When strawberries are in season, I buy them by the boxful, gorge like a bear, and freeze bagsful for another time.

240ml water
240ml skimmed milk
120ml egg substitute
60ml frozen white grape juice
1 medium banana
300g fresh or frozen strawberries
2 tbs cocoa powder

Banana Blueberry Bonanza

Of all the berries, blueberries have the highest antioxidant potential. Once again, whenever they're in season, I have my fill and freeze for the future.

240ml water
240ml skimmed milk
60ml frozen red grape juice concentrate (this goes well with all berry smoothies)
120ml egg substitute
2 medium bananas
200g fresh or 150g frozen blueberries (or more if you prefer, as I do)

Purple Cow

When I was small, my mum used to mix a glass of milk with grape juice, calling it a purple cow. This smoothie has all that flavour and more nutritional value.

243ml water
240ml skimmed milk
120ml egg substitute
90ml frozen red grape juice concentrate
175g seedless red or black grapes
1 medium banana

Chocolate Peanut Butter Cup

The authentic sweet confection is one of my favourites, but I avoid it because of the saturated fat content. So I came up with this smoothie to satisfy my craving. The peanut butter adds some healthy fat and the extra calories keep away the hunger pangs for a long time.

240ml water
240ml skimmed milk
1 medium banana
1 medium pear
120ml egg substitute
60ml frozen orange juice concentrate
2–3 tbsp peanut butter
2 tbsp honey
2 heaped tbsp cocoa powder

Melon Madness

This isn't really a smoothie so much as a 'fruit slurry'. Call it what you will, it's a cold, refreshing and nourishing drink during the summer melon season.

240ml water
200g cantaloupe chunks
200g honeydew melon chunks
200g seedless watermelon chunks
2 tbsp honey

Desserts and treats

Here are more opportunities to incorporate fruit into your diet in delicious ways far beyond simply gnawing on an apple or peeling a banana. Preparation is remarkably simple and takes little time.

Bananas Flambé without the Flame

 2 bananas sliced lengthways
 1 tbsp brown sugar
 1 tbsp soft margarine
 Low-fat vanilla ice cream

Melt the margarine in a frying pan on a low heat and add brown sugar. Stir until the sugar melts and blends with the margarine. Sauté and brown the bananas. Serve with a scoop of ice cream for each banana. Serves two.

The original recipe, which you can copy if you feel like getting fancy some evening, calls for adding a tablespoon of banana liqueur and a tablespoon of brandy to the melted margarine and sugar, heating, and then igniting with a match to yield a spectacular effect. If you'd like the taste of the liqueur and brandy without the flame, you can simply add them to the pan and heat for a while without igniting.

'Toffee Apples' on a Plate – not a Stick

 1 apple per person
 1 tbsp low-fat or fat-free caramel ice cream topping
 2 tbsp chopped walnuts

Slice the apple and place slices on a plate. Drizzle with the caramel topping. Top with the chopped walnuts.

Grilled Pineapple

Pineapple can be quite sharp, unless you happen to be enjoying it on a tropical island where the fruit grows and it's picked at its perfect ripeness. Heating the pineapple, in this case grilling it, breaks down the starch into natural sugars and releases a wonderfully sweet flavour.

 1 pineapple sliced into rings
 Maple syrup, honey or brown sugar

Arrange the pineapple slices on a grill pan and drizzle with your sweetener of choice. Grill until brown. You can also grill over barbecue coals.

Raspberries and Chambord Liqueur

This is an elegant dessert idea for entertaining. Serve each person a plate on which you place a small bowl of fresh, rinsed raspberries (best when in season), a spirit glass containing Chambord raspberry liqueur and a toothpick. Use the toothpick to pierce and pick up a raspberry to dip into the liqueur. You'll get raves for this no-effort presentation.

Mango with Sticky Rice

1 large mango, peeled and sliced, for two persons
200g cooked Japanese sticky rice, warm not hot

The short list above says it all. Just arrange the mango slices to one side of a small dessert plate and place the warm rice on the other. The combined tastes are marvellous. You may see this dessert on an expensive Thai restaurant menu.

Fruit and Cheese Platter

This is the ultimate continental dessert, enjoyed far more often by the French than more elaborate dishes. You need just a little of the strong-flavoured cheeses suggested here to offset the sweetness of the fruit. Some 15g of cheese has just over 4g of fat. This 'recipe' serves two.

1 apple
1 pear
175g grapes
30g blue, cheddar or brie cheese

Thinly slice the apple and pear and arrange half of each in fans on a platter with half the grapes and 15g of cheese. Try this with a glass of full-bodied red wine.

Peach Melba

Here's a flashback to the 1950s. If you're younger than 55 you may never have heard of it. Either way, just reading the following recipe is sure to rev up your taste buds.

> 70g raspberry jam
> 3 tbsp brown sugar
> 100ml water
> 4 large peaches, stoned, peeled and sliced (use fresh or frozen)
> 1 tsp lemon juice
> 350g fresh raspberries
> Low-fat vanilla ice cream

This is a variation on the classic recipe, eliminating the brandy added to the frying pan to flambé the dessert. You can do that if you wish, but it's really not necessary.

Combine the jam, sugar and water in a frying pan and simmer over a low heat for about 5 minutes or until syrupy. Add the peaches and cook for another 3–4 minutes, turning a few times until tender. Add the lemon juice and stir through.

Divide the cooked peaches on four plates and top with a small scoop of ice cream. Spoon the syrupy sauce over the peaches and ice cream. Top with raspberries.

Dawn's Gooey Chocolate Cake

My wife Dawn is a far better cake maker than I am, since she likes to follow recipes to the letter whereas I tend to wing it. Baking calls for strict adherence to directions. But this recipe is easy enough even for me to follow without messing it up. But it tastes better when Dawn makes this cake for me – it's the love factor. Beyond the sheer indulgence, you'll get the polyphenols of cocoa and the good fats, omega-3 fatty acids, of walnuts. Dawn modified this recipe from the original 1969 *Betty Crocker's Cookbook* that both of us use more than any other cookbook in our rather large library.

> 150g flour (use wholemeal to make it extra healthy)
> 200g granulated sugar
> 2 tbsp cocoa powder (not hot cocoa mix)
> 2 tsp baking powder
> ¼ tsp salt
> 100ml skimmed milk
> 2 tbsp soft margarine, melted but not hot
> 175g chopped walnuts
> 200g brown sugar
> 25g cocoa powder
> 400ml hot water

Preheat oven to 180°C/350°F/Gas 4. Blend flour, granulated sugar, the 2 tablespoons of cocoa powder, baking powder and salt in a mixing bowl. Add the milk and margarine and stir in the walnuts. Pour the mixture into an ungreased 20x20x5cm square cake tin. Mix the brown sugar and the 25g cocoa powder and sprinkle over the mixture in the cake tin. Pour the hot water over the mix. Bake for 45 minutes.

You'll wind up with a wonderful combination of cake and pudding. Cut the cake into squares for serving, topped with the pudding. We like to top it off with low-fat whipped cream or vanilla ice cream. Make this once and it'll become one of your favourites.

Chocolate Banana Pudding

Here's a dessert that combines the BP-lowering benefits of potassium in the banana with the polyphenols of cocoa.

Simply slice a ripe banana into instant or regular (cooked) fat-free chocolate pudding mix. Conversely, mix 2 heaped tablespoons of cocoa powder into fat-free pudding mix and slice in a banana.

BP-lowering Hot Cocoa

Ever since I learned the benefits of cocoa's polyphenols, I've been in the habit of sipping a cup of hot cocoa in the evening. It's a soothing, relaxing and healthy ritual before bedtime. The following recipe is for one mug/serving, but you can multiply it for more than one person.

Heat 240ml skimmed milk in the microwave. Put 2 tablespoons dark cocoa and 1 tablespoon sugar (or equivalent artificial sweetener) in a mug. Pour the heated milk into the mug and stir. Top the mug with a few mini-marshmallows for a treat.

Here are a few alternative hot cocoa flavours. Just add one of the following to the blend:

1 tbsp raspberry jam, 1 tbsp frozen red grape or orange juice concentrate, 1 tsp vanilla extract or 1 tsp instant coffee (decaf at bedtime). Or add a pinch of cinnamon or nutmeg or both.

New York Egg Cream

To the uninitiated, this beverage must contain egg and cream, right? Wrong. How it got its name is a matter of conjecture, but it's a delicious treat from Brooklyn and is served in delis throughout the US and elsewhere.

The original recipe calls for 2 tablespoons of chocolate syrup, 100ml of whole milk and 100ml of soda water. But I've modified that significantly to make an equally delicious alternative that packs more of cocoa's polyphenols and eliminates the sodium in the soda water.

In a large glass, mix 2 tablespoons chocolate syrup and 1 tablespoon cocoa powder until the cocoa is completely blended. Next add 120ml cold, skimmed milk and stir. Now add 120ml cold sparkling water followed by another 120ml cold milk. Stir gently to save the bubbles. Serve with ice cubes and sip through a straw for authenticity.

Chapter 18

Take the Pressure Off Your Heart

Whoops, I nearly forgot to mention the most important 'weapons' to lower blood pressure and prevent cardiovascular disease, heart attack and stroke. You've read about ways to cope with stress, lose weight, stop smoking cigarettes, become more physically active, improve your diet and counterbalance salt and sodium. You've learned about natural, safe and clinically documented supplements that can dramatically lower both systolic and diastolic blood pressure. Those supplements weren't even available when I was first inspired to write this book after studying newly published blood pressure guidelines in 2003. So what's missing?

If some company could bottle the following ingredients, which virtually guarantee success in blood pressure control and heart disease prevention, doctors worldwide would write the prescription and the company would make countless millions of dollars, euros, pounds and yen. But no one ever will because those truly secret ingredients can be found only in your own heart and soul. They are motivation and commitment.

It has now been well over two decades since that cardiac surgeon told me that the second bypass operation I needed might kill me, leaving my children without their dad. If some mysterious supernatural being came into my apartment that day when I wept at the thought of my wife having to tell little Ross and Jenny that Daddy's never coming home from the hospital, I would have jumped at any deal on offer. I would have gladly accepted postponing death until the day they went off to college and were more or less on their own. Those kids were my motivation and the source of my continued commitment through the years.

Of course, it turns out I didn't have to sign that sort of contract, and it's a good thing that I didn't. I've lived to see Ross and Jenny grow up into fine young adults. They're well on their way to productive careers. I've outlived my father by many years. My cardiologist calls my test reports superb. I never expected to live this long.

But now I've got greedy! Life has never been better, never sweeter. I love my wife Dawn and we're looking forward to growing older together and enjoying some of the rewards of decades of hard work, such as travel, and savouring the simple joys of reading a book, watching the sun set and marvelling at the beauty of a flower or a bird or a mountain. Ross and Jenny still like to ask my advice on personal and professional matters. And I want to be around for that day when my first grandchild is born and I get to hold him or her in my arms, to witness all those wonderful stages of childhood, and dole out all the love I have in my heart. Lord, how I wish my dad had had that chance. Sadly he did not, but I do. The realisation for those hopes and dreams in the future, sharing life with my wonderful family, remain my motivation and commitment.

But enough about me! What about you? What are the reasons for your motivation and commitment to health? What are your reasons for taking the pressure off your heart by lowering your blood pressure? What will inspire you to take that brisk walk when you'd rather watch TV? To make food choices based on reasons other than taste alone? To lose those extra pounds and put out that last cigarette? To religiously take those supplements? Only you have the incredible power to choose a long and healthy life. Or should I say to *work* for that life.

Most men and women never really stop, as the old proverb goes, to smell the roses. They don't even bother to look at them. Close your eyes for a moment. Think about all the true joys in your life: your family, your career, your hobbies, your religious beliefs. Do you love to fish, to go rambling, to cook? What will be *your* motivation?

Even more than when I first began to write this book, I now know that the programme in these pages really works. Readers of my quarterly publication *The Diet-Heart Newsletter* had an advance opportunity to try the programme for themselves before the book came even close to publication. Every time I got a report of success from them, I felt not selfish pride but gratitude that I could share this information. Doctors who have incorporated the programme into their clinical practices tell me over and over about how their patients' have benefited.

But no programme will do any good until you make it a part of your own life. No drug company or supplement maker will put motivation and commitment into pills or tablets or capsules for you to swallow.

A frequent theme in literature and in the movies involves a person seeing the world after his or her death. Think Dickens's *A Christmas Carol*. Now think about the world without you. Imagine the tears of your loved ones. Picture yourself not being able to do all the things you've wanted to do. Four decades later, I still miss my father. My wife and children would certainly miss me. And many would miss you.

The time to live is now. The time to ensure a long, healthy, happy life is now. Find that motivation in your heart, your inner self, to take the pressure off your heart – starting today. For tomorrow and tomorrow and tomorrow. Join me in the celebration of heart health!

References

Chapter 1
Heart, December 2005
Hypertension Management Guide for Doctors, 2004, Heart
    Foundation of Australia
British Medical Journal, June 2001
Circulation, 18 June 2002
Stroke, February 2006
Proceedings of the American College of Cardiology, March
    2006
American Journal of Kidney Diseases, March 2003
American Journal of Medicine, February 2006
Annals of Family Medicine, July–August 2005
The Lancet, 17 November 2001
New England Journal of Medicine, 1 November 2001
Journal of the American Medical Association (JNC-7 Report),
    21 May 2003
New England Journal of Medicine, 15 March 2006
American Journal of Medicine, February 2006
Annals of Internal Medicine, 5 April 2006
Journal of the American Medical Association, 14 May 2003
New England Journal of Medicine, 20 April 2006

Chapter 2
Journal of the American Medical Association, 31 May 2003
Archives of Internal Medicine, 11 July 2005
Circulation, 18 March 2003
American Journal of Hypertension, 4 February 2004
Hypertension, 30 December 2005

Chapter 3

Journal of the American Medical Association, 5 May 2004

Proceedings of the American Society of Nephrology Annual Meeting, November 2005

National High Blood Pressure Education Program Working Group on High Blood Pressure in Children and Adolescents, 2004

Pediatrics, June 2004

Circulation, 21 November 2005

American Heart Association: Heart Facts, 2003

Medscape Cardiology, Hypertension Highlights, 11 November 2003

Circulation, 30 January 2006

American College of Cardiology Annual Scientific Sessions, 2004

Journal Watch Cardiology, 23 November 2005

Medscape Cardiology, 5 April 2005

Journal of the American Medical Association, 27 July 2005

Stroke, May 2006

Chapter 4

Diabetes & Cardiovascular Disease Review: Hypertension in Diabetes, a publication of the American Diabetes Association/American College of Cardiology, 2002.

British Journal of Diabetes and Vascular Disease, March 2006

Diabetes Care, March 2004

Life Sciences, October 2004

Circulation, 3 February 2004

Circulation, 27 March 2006

Medscape Cardiology, 19 October 2005

Journal of the American Medical Association, 8 October 2003

Hypertension, March 2006

Chapter 5

Journal of the American Medical Association, 4 January 2006

The Lancet, 5 November 2005

American Journal of Clinical Nutrition, March 2004

American Journal of Hypertension, May 2004

Annals of Internal Medicine, 3 January 2006

Archives of Internal Medicine, 13 June 2005

Medical Journal of Australia, November–December 2003

American Journal of Clinical Nutrition, June 2005

Food Values of Portions Commonly Used, Jean A. T. Pennington, Lippincott, Williams & Wilkins, 17th edition

Environmental Nutrition, February 2006

Circulation, 31 January 2006

Chapter 6

Annals of Internal Medicine, April 2002

Preventive Medicine, September 2005

The Lancet, 8 October 2005

Circulation, 26 July 2005

Circulation, 18 September 2001

Circulation, 18 February 2003

Chapter 7

Stroke, 3 August 2001

Circulation, 20 May 2002

American Journal of Hypertension, 16 July 2001

Journal of Clinical Hypertension, 4 August 2004

Circulation, 23 March 2004

Proceedings of the Scientific Sessions of the American Heart Association, November 2005

British Medical Journal (Online First), 19 January 2006

Medical Journal of Australia (Stress Position Statement), 2003

Chapter 8
Action on Smoking and Health (ASH) website
(www.ash.org.uk), September 2006

Chapter 9
Sodium
Journal of Clinical Hypertension, 14 July 2004
British Medical Journal, 21 September 2002
Hypertension, 7 June 1995
The Lancet, 14 January 2006
Australian Heart Foundation, 'Salt and Hypertension',
February 2002

Potassium
Hypertension, 12 April 2005
Food Values of Portions Commonly Used, Jean Pennington,
Lippincott 2005
Annals of Internal Medicine, 15 July 1991
Proceedings of the American Heart Association, November
1994
British Journal of Nutrition, July 2003
Hypertension, 24 January 2005

Calcium
Proceedings of the American Heart Association, November
1992
American Journal of Hypertension, 24 October 2003

Magnesium
American Journal of Hypertension, 21 August 2002
American Journal of Cardiology, 10 October 2003
Medscape Medical News, 8 January 2004
Circulation, 4 April 2006

Chapter 10

Hypertension, 23 January 2006
American Journal of Geriatric Cardiology, June 2005
Archives of Internal Medicine, 22 March 2004
Circulation, 6 September 2005
The Lancet, 3 December 2005
American Journal of Hypertension, 19 October 2005
British Medical Journal, 20 January 2006
Stroke, 18 January 2006
Stroke, 25 January 2006
National Heart Foundation of Australia, 'Non-drug
   management of hypertension', September 2004
American Journal of Hypertension, February 2006

Chapter 11

Hypertension, January 2006
American Journal of Clinical Nutrition, November 2005
New England Journal of Medicine, 22 September 2005
Journal of the American Medical Association, 16 November
   2005
Archives of Internal Medicine, 14 November 2005
*Proceedings of the American Heart Association Annual
   Scientific Sessions*, November 2005
European Heart Journal, September 2005
Circulation, November 1999
Stroke, January 1997
Circulation, June 1997
American Journal of Clinical Nutrition, April 2006

Chapter 12
Effects of diet on blood pressure
The Lancet, 28 January 2006
American Journal of Clinical Nutrition, February 2006
Journal of Clinical Hypertension, April 2005
Diabetes Care, December 2005

Archives of Internal Medicine, 9 January 2006
Hypertension, 19 May 2003

Chocolate
Hypertension, 18 July 2005

Coffee and tea
Journal of the American Medical Association,
    9 November 2005
Journal of the American College of Cardiology,
    17 January 2006
Archives of Internal Medicine, 26 July 2004

Omega-3 fatty acids
Circulation, 19 August 2003
American Heart Association Scientific Statement,
    19 November 2002
American Journal of Clinical Nutrition, January 2003
Circulation, 27 September 2005
New England Journal of Medicine, 28 November 2000

Chapter 13
Acupuncture
Abstracts from the American Heart Association Scientific
    Sessions, 2005

Arginine
Journal of the American College of Nutrition, February 2002
American Journal of Nutrition, March 2000
Alternative Medicine Review, March 2002
Journal of Nutrition, December 2000
International Journal of Cardiology, February 2002

Aspirin
Proceedings of the Annual Conference on Arteriosclerosis,

Thrombosis, and Vascular Biology, 2004
Journal of the American Medical Association,
    18 January 2006
New England Journal of Medicine, 7 March 2005

Breathing
Medscape Cardiology, 25 July 2002
High-blood-pressure-help.com

Co-enzyme Q10
Naturaldatabase.com, February 2003
Pharmacotherapy, May 2001
Journal of Human Hypertension, February 1999
Southern Medical Journal, July 2001

Eye tests
British Journal of Ophthalmology, March 2005
British Journal of Ophthalmology, August 2005
Hypertension, August 2004

Fermented milk
American Journal of Hypertension, January 2006

Fish oil
Naturaldatabase.com, February 2003
Alternative Medical Review, April 2001
Prostaglandins, Leucotrienes and Essential Fatty Acids,
    January 1999
Medscape Cardiology, June 2004

Folic acid
American Journal of Clinical Nutrition, July 2005
*Proceedings of the American Heart Association Council for
    High Blood Pressure Research*, 2004
Stroke, September 2005

Garlic

Naturaldatabase.com, February 2003
Archives of Internal Medicine, April 2001
Journal of Hypertension, March 1994
Journal of Nutrition (Supplement), 2001

Herbs

Phytotherapy Research, January 2002
MayoClinic.com, November 2005

Laughter

Heart, February 2006

Loneliness

Psychology and Aging, March 2006

Melatonin

Hypertension, January 2004
American Journal of Hypertension, December 2005

Music

Heart, October 2005
British Medical Journal, September 2001

Over-the-counter and prescription-only medication

Archives of Internal Medicine, August 2005
American Journal of Medicine, September 2005
Consumerlab.com, November 2005
MayoClinic.com, November 2005
Heart Foundation (Australia): Non-Drug Management
    of Hypertension, September 2004

Sleep disorders

Hypertension, 4 May 2006
Current Hypertension Reports, October 2003

Current Cardiology Reports, November 2005
Hypertension, 3 February 2006
Hypertension, 3 April 2006

Vitamin supplements
Naturaldatabase.com, February 2003
Alternative Medicine Review, April 2001
The Lancet, December 1999

Chapter 14

Arginine
Journal of the American Medical Association, 4 January 2006
Recent Progress in Medicine (Italian), October 2005
American Journal of Cardiology, 10 October 2005
Canadian Journal of Physiology and Pharmacology,
    August–September 2005
British Journal of Pharmacology, January 2006
Vascular Medicine, November 2005
Vascular Medicine, July 2005
Alternative Medicine Review, January 2005
Circulation (Abstracts of the American Heart Association
    Scientific Sessions), November 2006
Personal Correspondence: Dr Lance Gould, University of
    Texas

Grape seed extract
American Journal of Clinical Nutrition (Supplement),
    January 2005
Abstracts, 219th American Chemical Society National
    Meeting, March 2000
American Journal of Clinical Nutrition, May 2002
Abstracts, Experimental Biology Conference, April 2005
Environmental Nutrition, May 2004
Chemical Innovation, September 2000

Circulation, 18 June 2002

Journal of Medicinal Food, 1 November 2001

Abstracts, 225th American Chemical Society National
Meeting, March 2006

European Journal of Clinical Pharmacology, February 2006

Bottom Line Health, January 2004

Lycopene and tomato extract

Biochemistry and Biophysics Research Communications, 28
April 1997

American Heart Journal, January 2006

Abstracts, American Chemical Society Annual Meeting,
March 2006

American Journal of Clinical Nutrition (Supplement),
January 2005

Pycnogenol

Life Sciences, June 2004

Nutrition Research, September 2001

Evidence-Based Integrative Medicine, August 2003

European Bulletin of Drug Research, July 1999

Journal of Cardiovascular Pharmacology, March 1998

Chocolate and cocoa

American Journal of Clinical Nutrition, January 2005

Hypertension, August 2005

Proceedings of the National Academy of Sciences, 24 January
2006

Pharmaceutical Business Review, March 2006

Archives of Internal Medicine, 27 February 2006

Chapter 15

New England Journal of Medicine, 20 January 2000

Journal of the American Medical Association, September
2002

Journal of the American Medical Association, 21 May 2003
The Lancet, 6 November 2004
The Lancet, 10 September 2005
Pharmacotherapy, November 2005
Journal of Hypertension, June 2003
Circulation, 2 May 2006
Medscape Cardiology internet search
American Heart Association internet search
American College of Cardiology internet search

Index

lumen, 199, 215
lunch, 67, 179
Lyc-O-Mato, 231–4, 267
lycopene, 231–2, 267

M
ma huang, 208
mackerel, 185
magnesium, 9, 54–5, 142–4, 202
  sources, 144
  supplements, 142, 144, 265
male impotence, 220–21
mango with sticky rice, 298
margarine, 159–60
marital relationships, poor, 98–9
masked hypertension (MH), 30–31
meats, 63, 71, 75, 158, 160, 178
  organic, 162
media, 214
meditation, 106–7
Mediterranean diet, 135, 160, 172,
  175, 178, 180, 188
Mediterranean salad, 272
Mega-Natural BP, 229–31, 238,
  267
melatonin, 7, 205–6
melon and avocado salad, 273
menopause, 43, 165
mental stress, 101–3
metabolic equivalent (MET), 82–4
  of common activities, 91–2
metabolic syndrome, 54, 144, 149,
  229
methyldopa, 255
micelles, 161, 162
milk, fermented, 198–9
mind/body connection, 93–109
mindfulness, 106–7
minestrone soup, 277
Minoxidil, 255–6
moderation, 133–5, 174, 184
  alcohol consumption, 150–51
monounsaturated fats, 160, 174
muscles, 75–6, 86, 169–70, 195–6
  cramps, 20, 143
music, 207

N
naproxen, 208
nebivolol, 219

niacin, 163–6, 168, 170, 221–2,
  266
  sustained-release, 165, 222
niacinamide, 166
NiaSpan, 166
nicotine, 117
  replacement, 120–21
nitric oxide (NO), 205, 211,
  217–21, 224, 228, 235–6, 241,
  266
  production, 53
noradrenaline, 102, 205
nosebleeds, 20
nutrition, 63–4
nuts, 159, 175, 186, 191

O
oat bran, 4, 8, 161, 168
obesity, 3, 43, 57–77, 263
  among black people, 18
  hypertension and, 18–19
oils, 63, 160, 189
  partially hydrogenated, 159,
  174
olive oil, 160, 175, 178, 266
omega-3 fatty acids, 159, 174–5,
  177, 184–7, 199, 266
Omron HEM-737 Intellisense, 33,
  263
oral contraceptives, 43, 209
over-the-counter drugs, 207–9
overweight, 3, 35, 57–77, 263
oxygen, maximum volume of, 83

P
painkillers, 208
palm kernel oils, 158
paracetamol, 208
parathyroid hormone, 141
peach Melba, 299
peanut oil, 160
pedometers, 89–90, 264
peppers: sautéed onions and, 285
  tri-colour roasted salad, 272
Perfusia-SR, 222, 225
perspiration, excessive, 20
physical activity, 19, 178, 264
  advantages of, 85–7
  importance, 78–92
  taking baby steps, 89–90